Pictures Through Dementia

VOLUME 4

Pictures Through Dementia: Volume 4

Copyright ©2021

ISBN # 978-1-7370685-2-5

Design by Deborah Perdue of Illumination Graphics
www.illuminationgraphics.com

DEDICATION

All credit to the Creator – the Forgiver
and the Miracle Maker

And pastors Tom, Tyrone, Mark, Phil, Bruce, Paula and the
dementia players: Irwin, Grant, Chavis, Downtown, Coo,
Theo, Emil, Alton, Tyon, Richard, Lisa, Soukups and Doc
Team Leader Sonia Delgado, with Alia and Ariel, Kayla and
Sara, Ms. Fauci, Mr. Cheatle and and Don Dolde

Gratitude to Christine Bryant, Kate Swaffer, Teepa Snow, and
the family at Dementia Alliance International

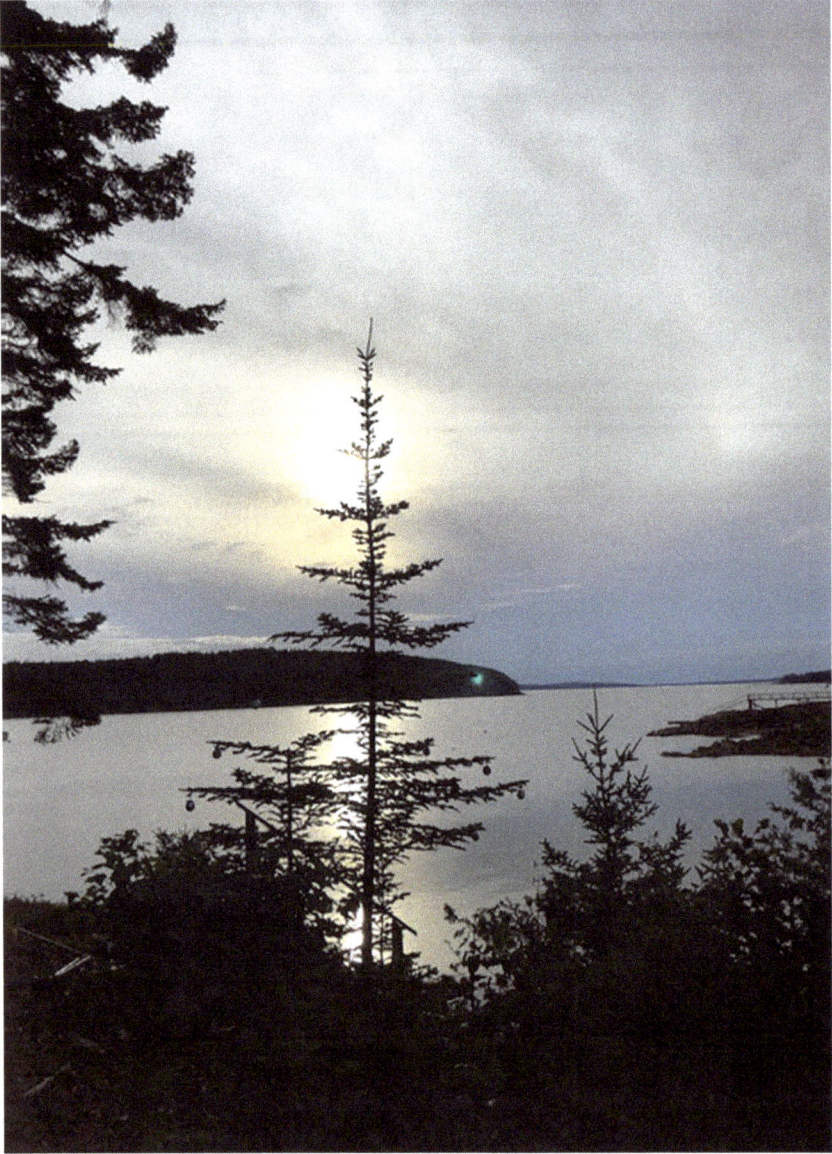

INTRODUCTION

The idea of this book is to educate, of course,

and to show the

progression of dementia.

This compilation of pictures is my way of saying goodbye

to the memories,

and to honor them in thanks to the Divine.

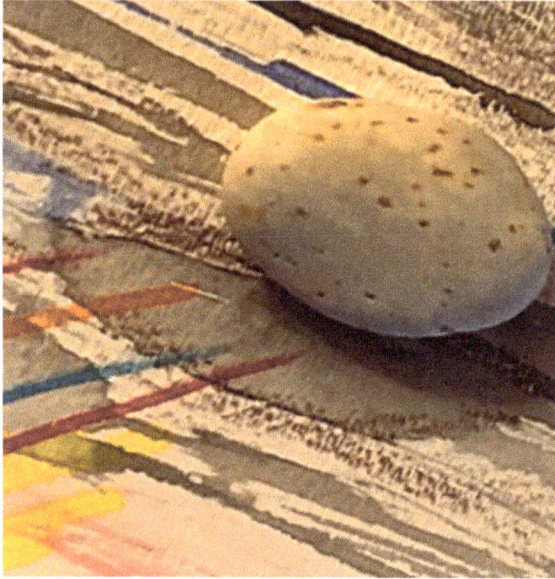

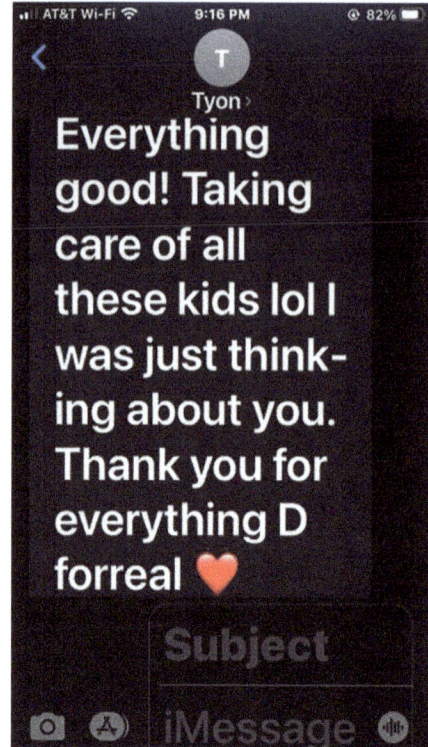

June 2021

I guess this dementia dude ought to have figured, but I recently became aware that regular people are disquieted when we have our more regular-person moments of acuity. Concerning, really. A sign perhaps that the caregiving is suspect.

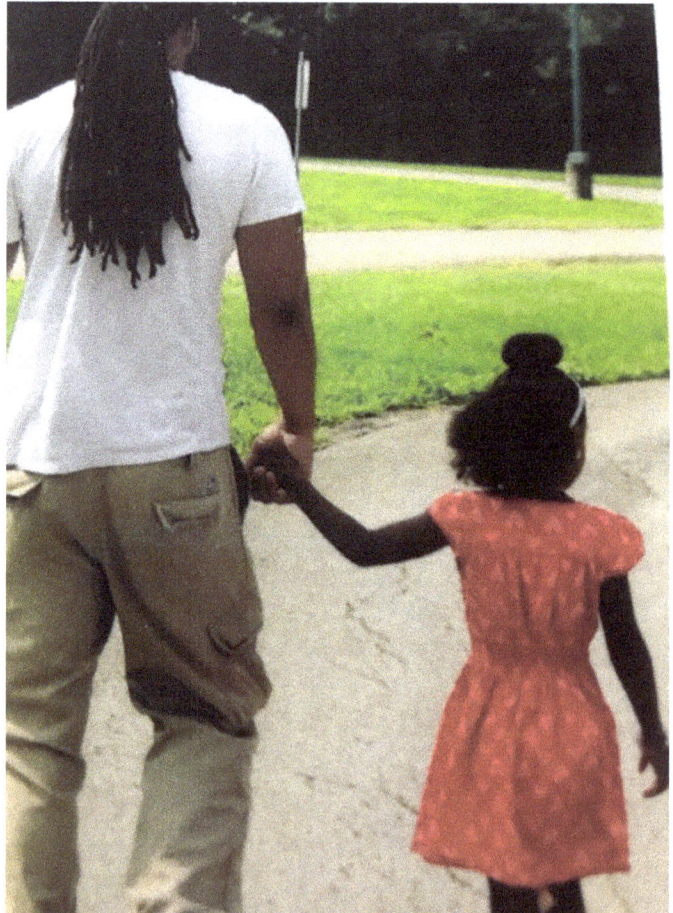

November 2020

I'm sureish I'm not the first to say that the simple difference between a faulty memory (age related or not) and us having a dementiafried memory is that it does us no good to search for the lost item or thought. Oh, you might find it sometimes, but it's rarely worth the effort.

2

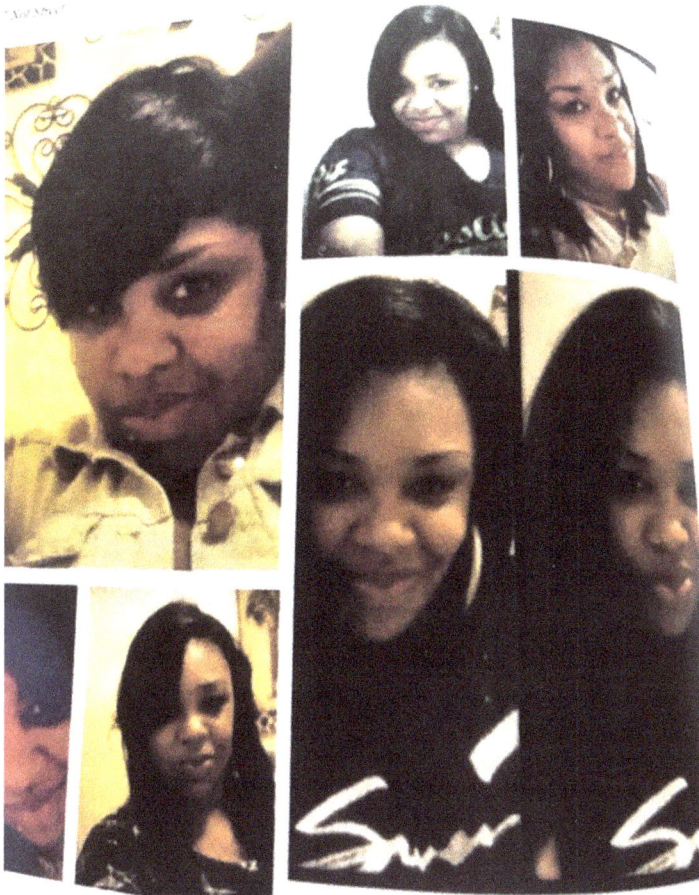

PLEASE BE PATIENT

The person I am with has dementia and:

* may not remember what you said.

* may repeat questions.

* may have difficulty speaking.

* may get scared easily.

Please speak clearly, use eye contact and a soft tone of voice.

Thank You
Alzheimer's New Jersey

"Yesterday I was clever so I wanted to change the world.
Today I am wise so I want to change myself."
Rumi

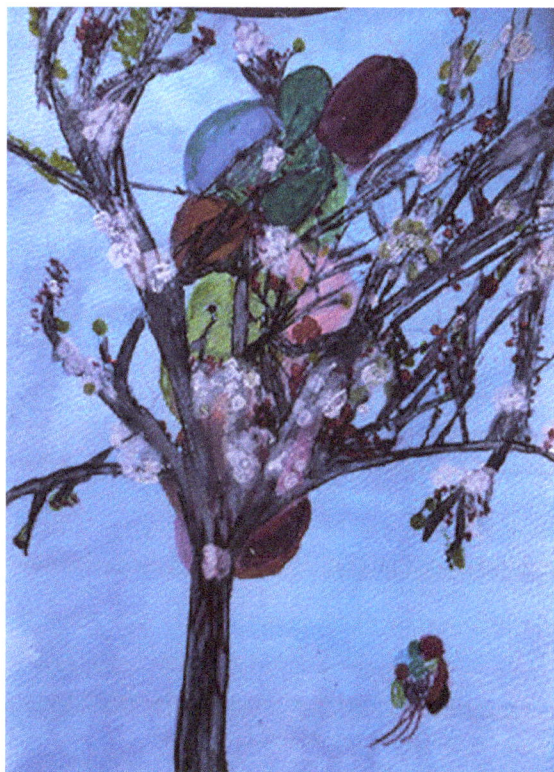

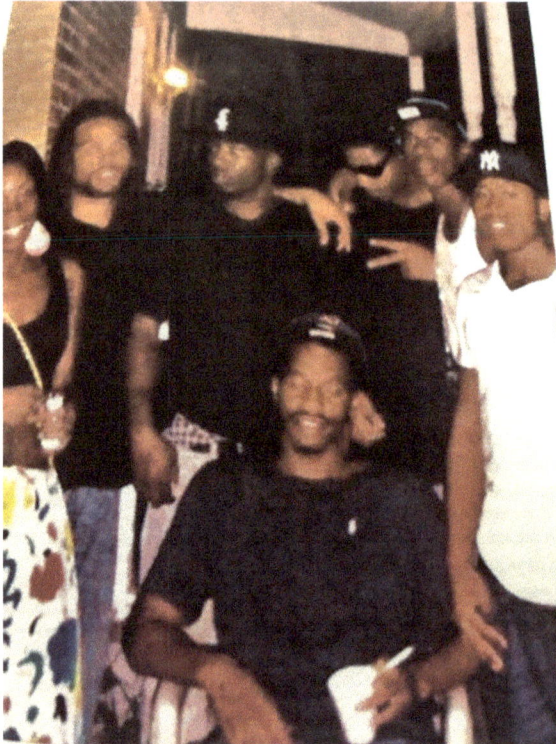

Note to Dementia Self:

Newish symptoms:
memories, dreams, and here and now
morphing together.

Sounds feel random and difficult to discern
their meanings, location, or volume.

All interesting after the trust in all is put away
as "the old way."

I guess it comes down that the relationship between regulars and us demented must be reciprocal and based on the verse, "be patient and bear with one another in love."

Christen Bryden was my first dementia hero; a trusting light at the end of the tunnel. I think I misspelled her first name (a bit dementiafried) I believe we should ask the Alzheimer's Association to unify with us folks and honor a true wisdom giver. Christine Bryden Day on the same day as they celebrate the Longest Day (which tires me out just thinking about it). Thoughts?

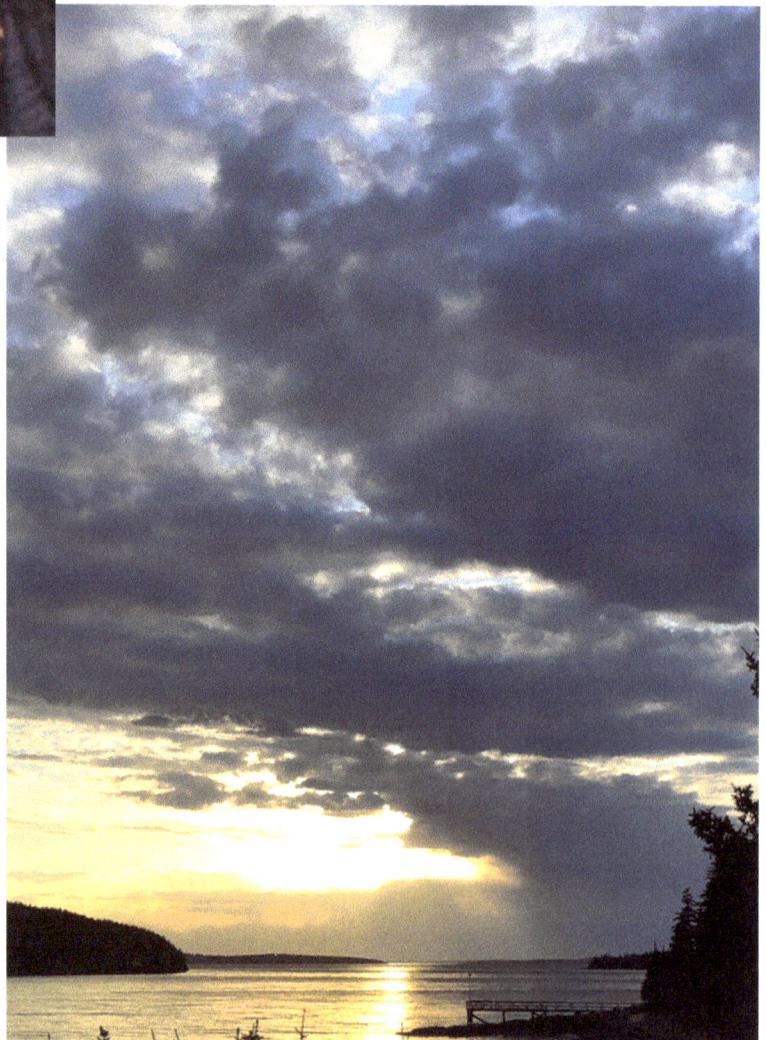

Just because our cognition is mushy does not mean our spirit is.

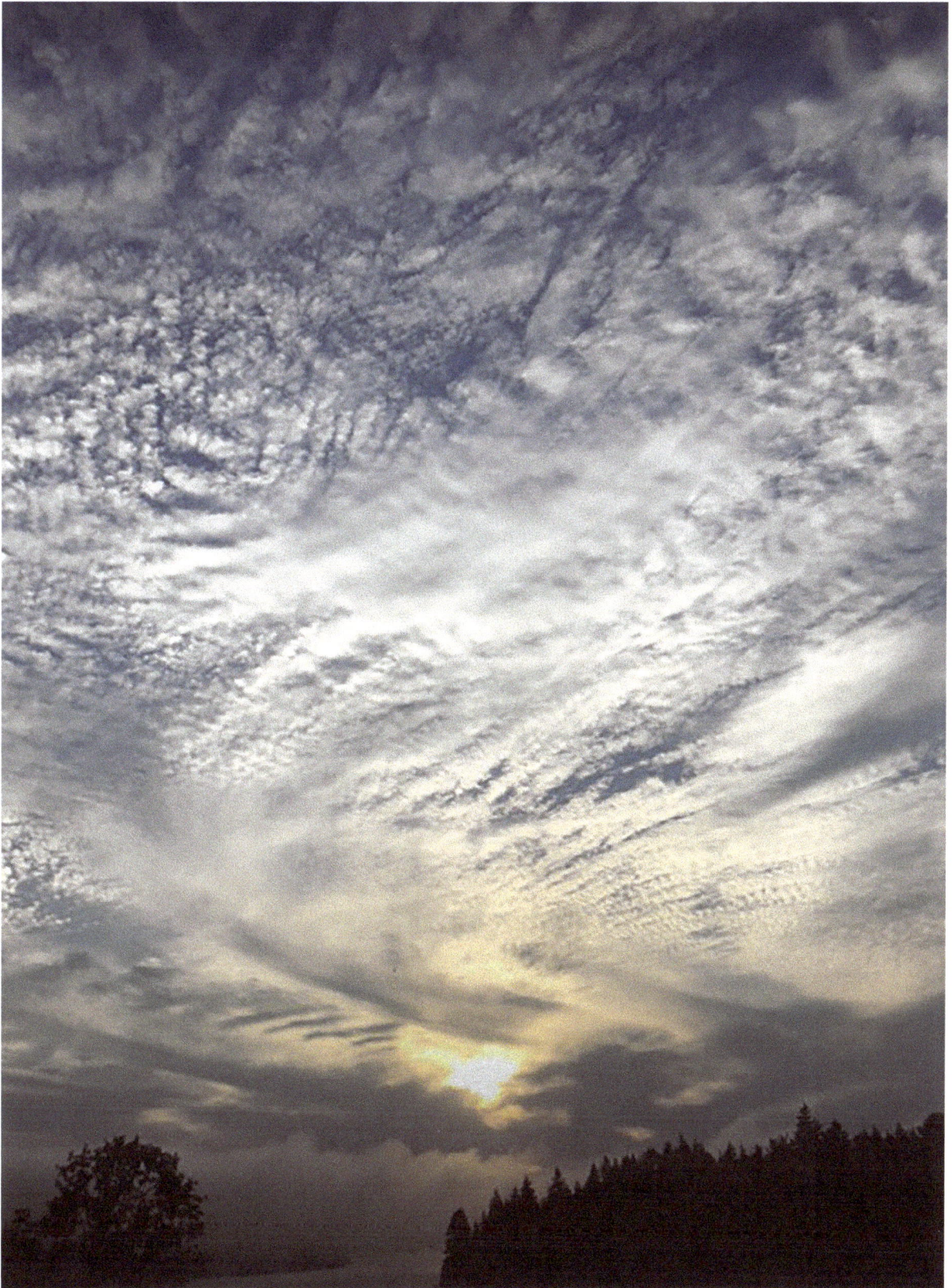

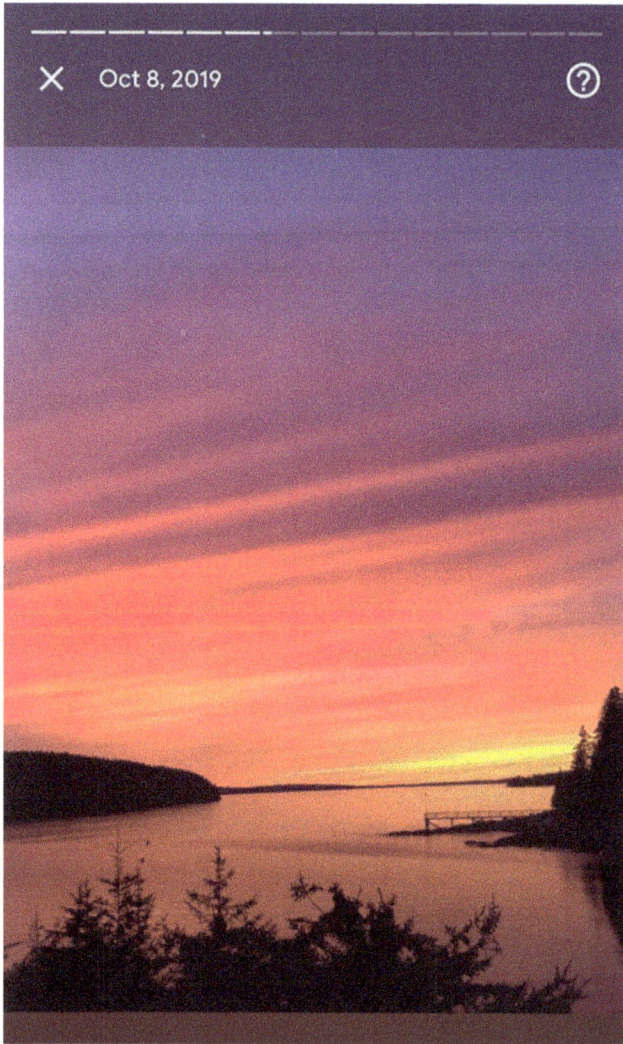

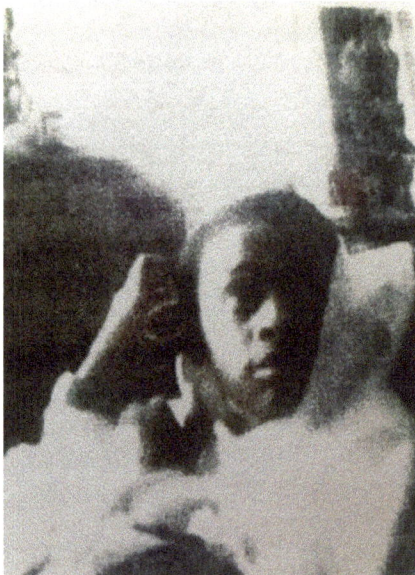

"Evolutionarily, we're always concerned with what's not right. That's what makes gratefulness delightfully subversive."
—Dale Biron

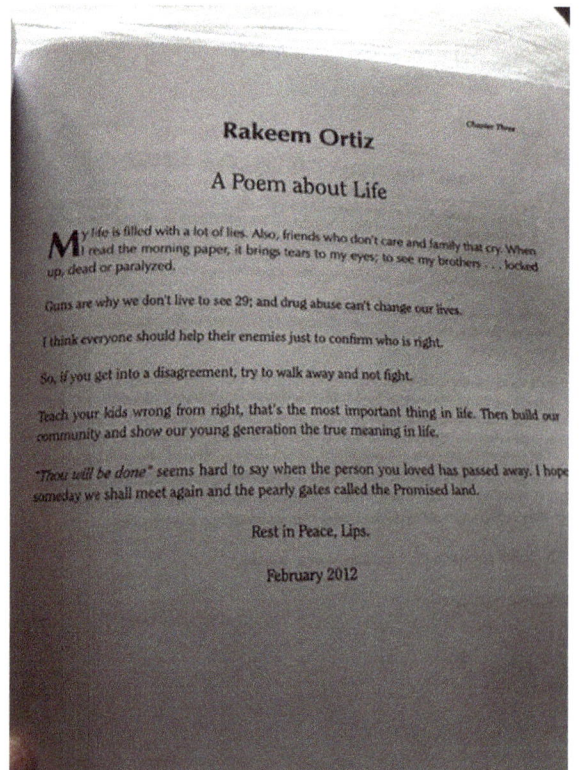

Rakeem Ortiz

Chapter Three

A Poem about Life

My life is filled with a lot of lies. Also, friends who don't care and family that cry. When I read the morning paper, it brings tears to my eyes; to see my brothers . . . locked up, dead or paralyzed.

Guns are why we don't live to see 29; and drug abuse can't change our lives.

I think everyone should help their enemies just to confirm who is right.

So, if you get into a disagreement, try to walk away and not fight.

Teach your kids wrong from right, that's the most important thing in life. Then build our community and show our young generation the true meaning in life.

"Thou will be done" seems hard to say when the person you loved has passed away. I hope someday we shall meet again and the pearly gates called the Promised land.

Rest in Peace, Lips.

February 2012

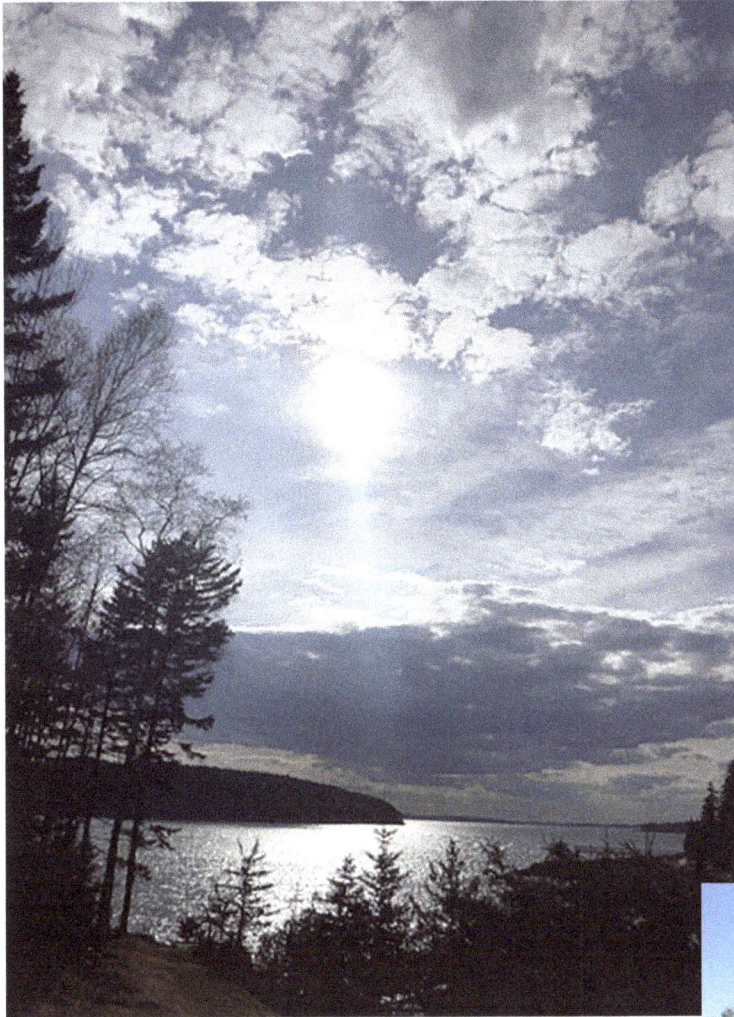

For you regular persons who are just beginning to learn about us dementia folk, it is a DEMENTIA VIOLATION TO EXPECT A JOLLY QUICK ANSWER AFTER ASKING US "Well, what did you do today?" Don't be a conversation fascist.

Dementia Tidbit: Casually and with no wrong intent, when you interrupt a dementia person

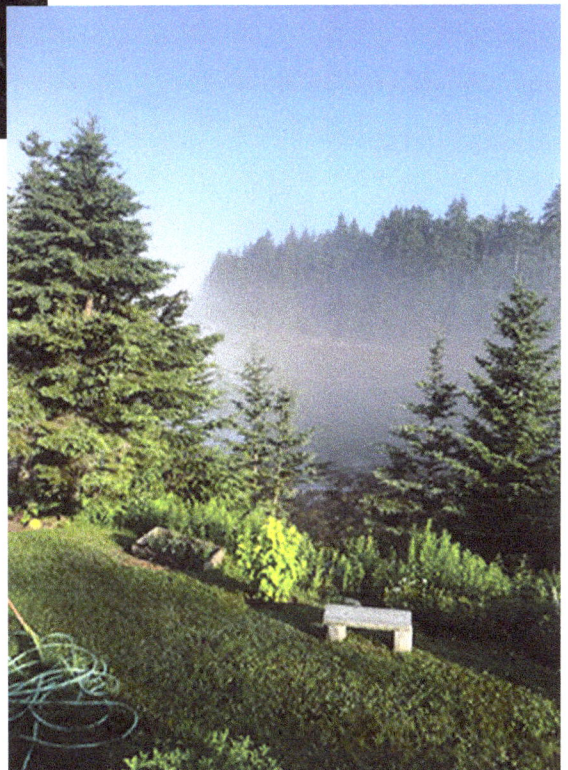

while they are speaking is like throwing a cherry bomb (fireworks) in our lap. Don't be a conversation fascist.

Dementia Alert: A recent study has given us hope after so many years of searching for a dementia cure. Well, maybe it will, partially, although the results are encouraging. We will now study . . . oh yes, any side effects. Celebrating too soon.

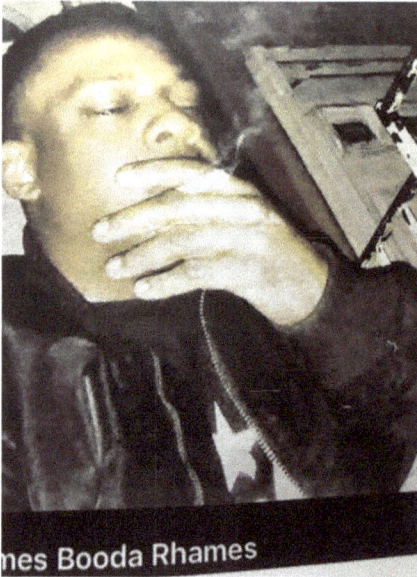

mes Booda Rhames

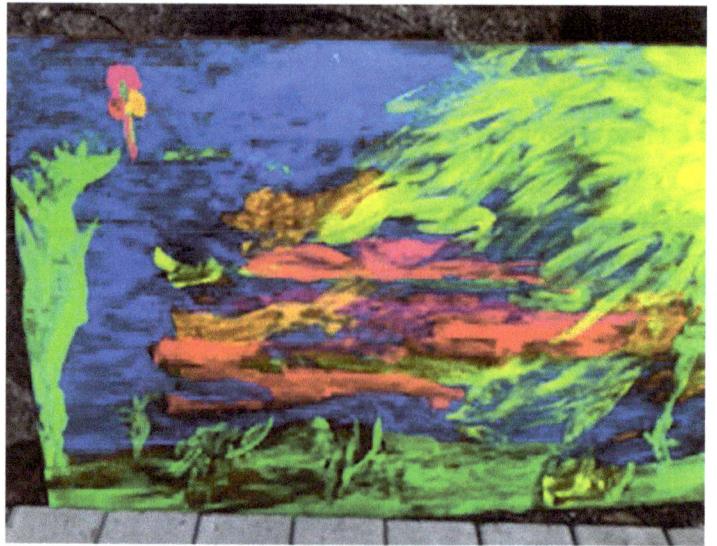

Dementia folks often spend our early years chasing diagnoses and cures. It's a bumpy time. Teepa Snow taught me how to discern my own dementia. Thankful.

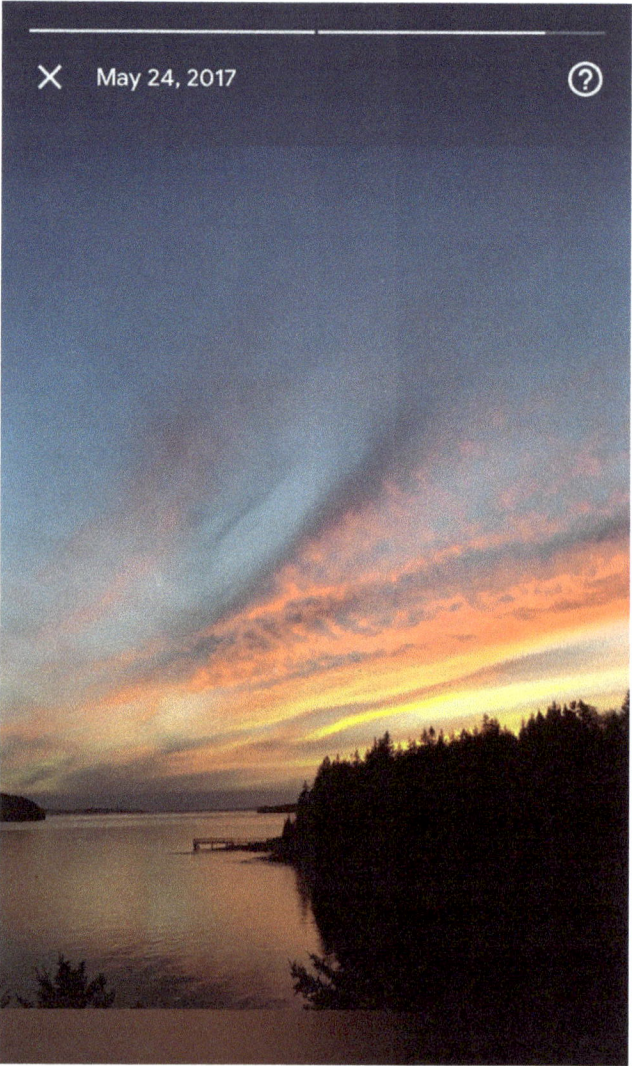

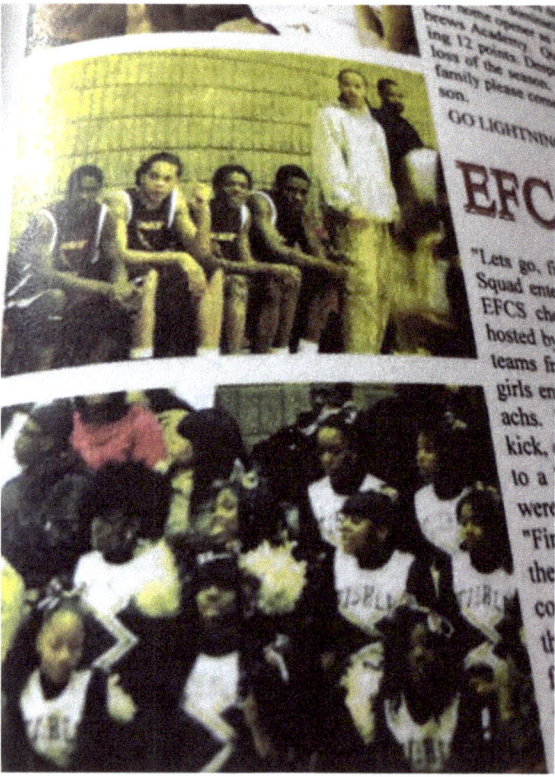

May 24, 2017

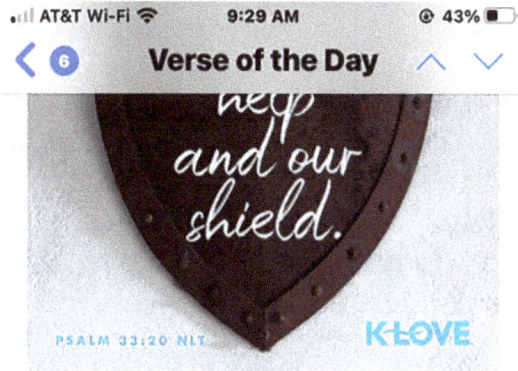

05/25/2021

We put our hope in the LORD. He is our help and our shield.

Psalm 33:20 (NLT) Read Full Chapter

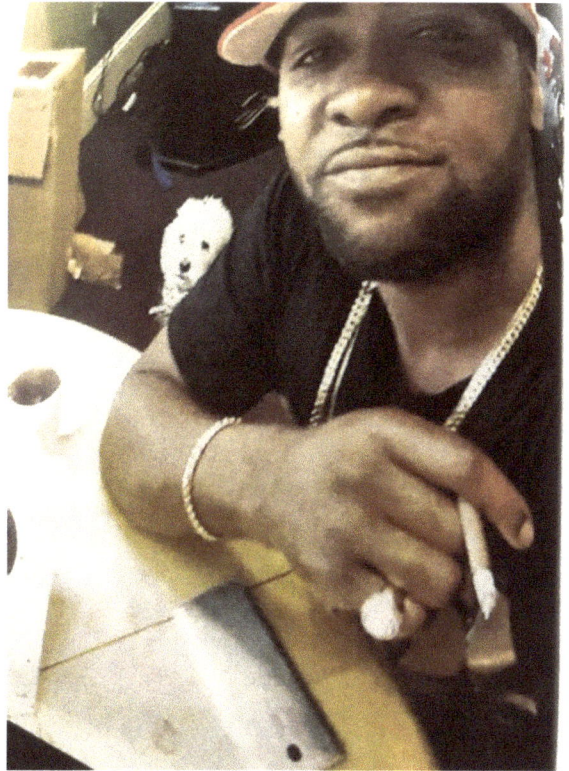

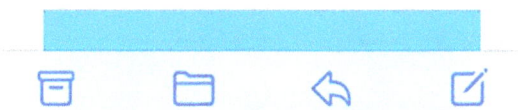

God, through my dementia, is cleaning the sludge from my soul.

Harry Johns, the self-proclaimed "global leader" of the Alzheimer's Association should resign. Join the demand.

God is often just a side hustle to dementia. Dementia should be a side hustle to God for us.

Dementia Dude taking photo ➜

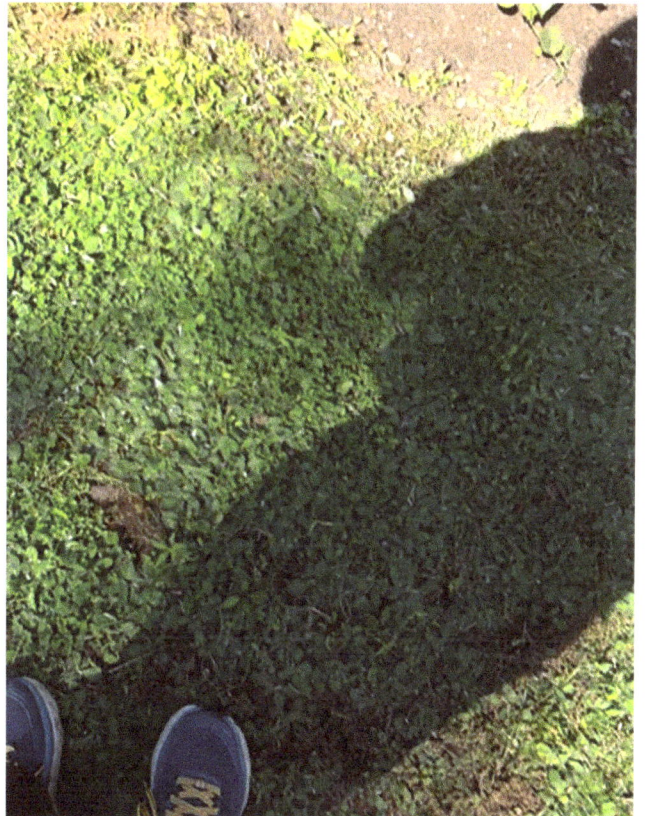

9

April 2021

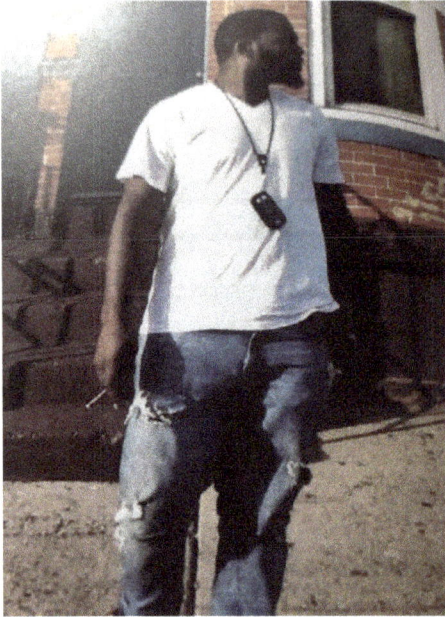

In the dementia world, it can get lonely like the regular world, but different. They have their own struggles; they have their own worlds. Not to mention ours is tough to navigate; not to mention our world keeps changing from a dementia perspective. The grace we desperately need is the same grace you need in sorting out us time surfers.

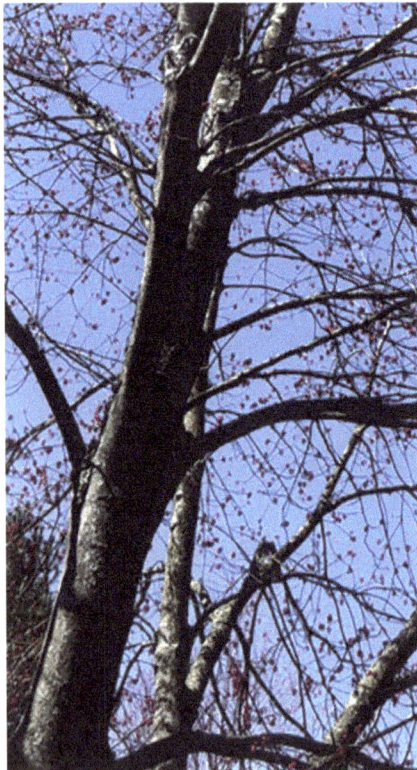

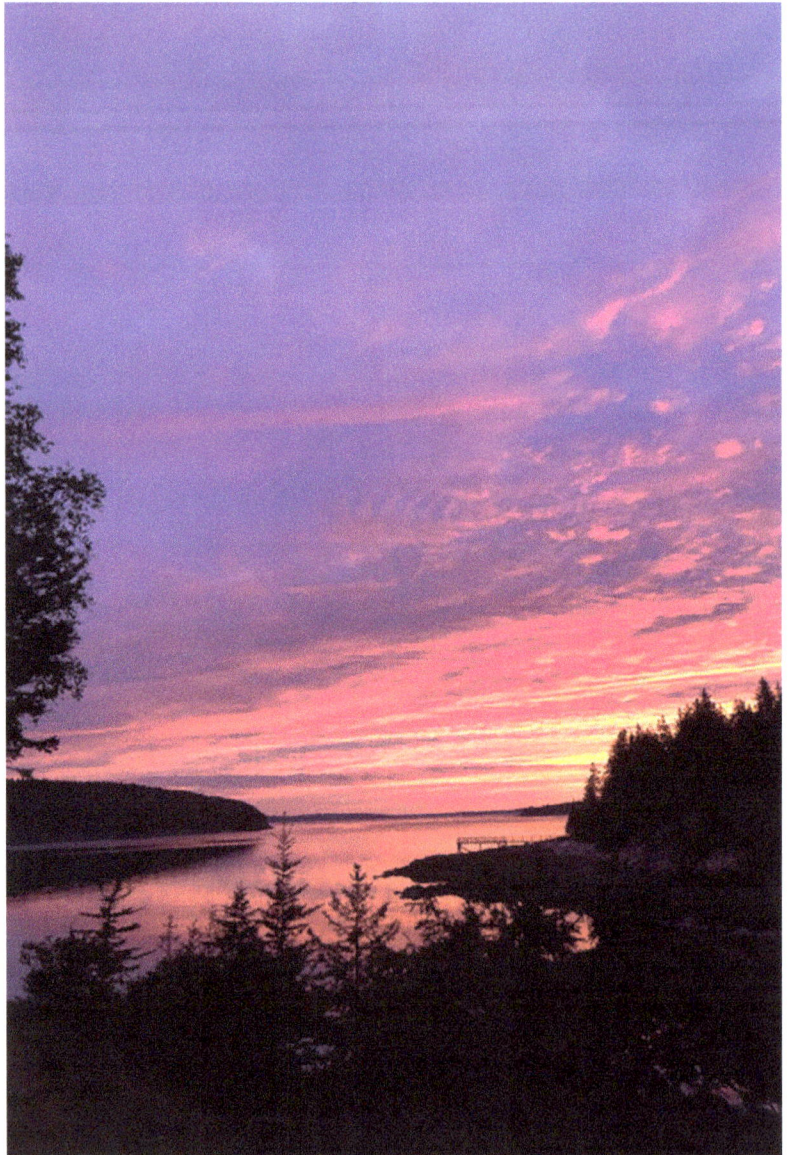

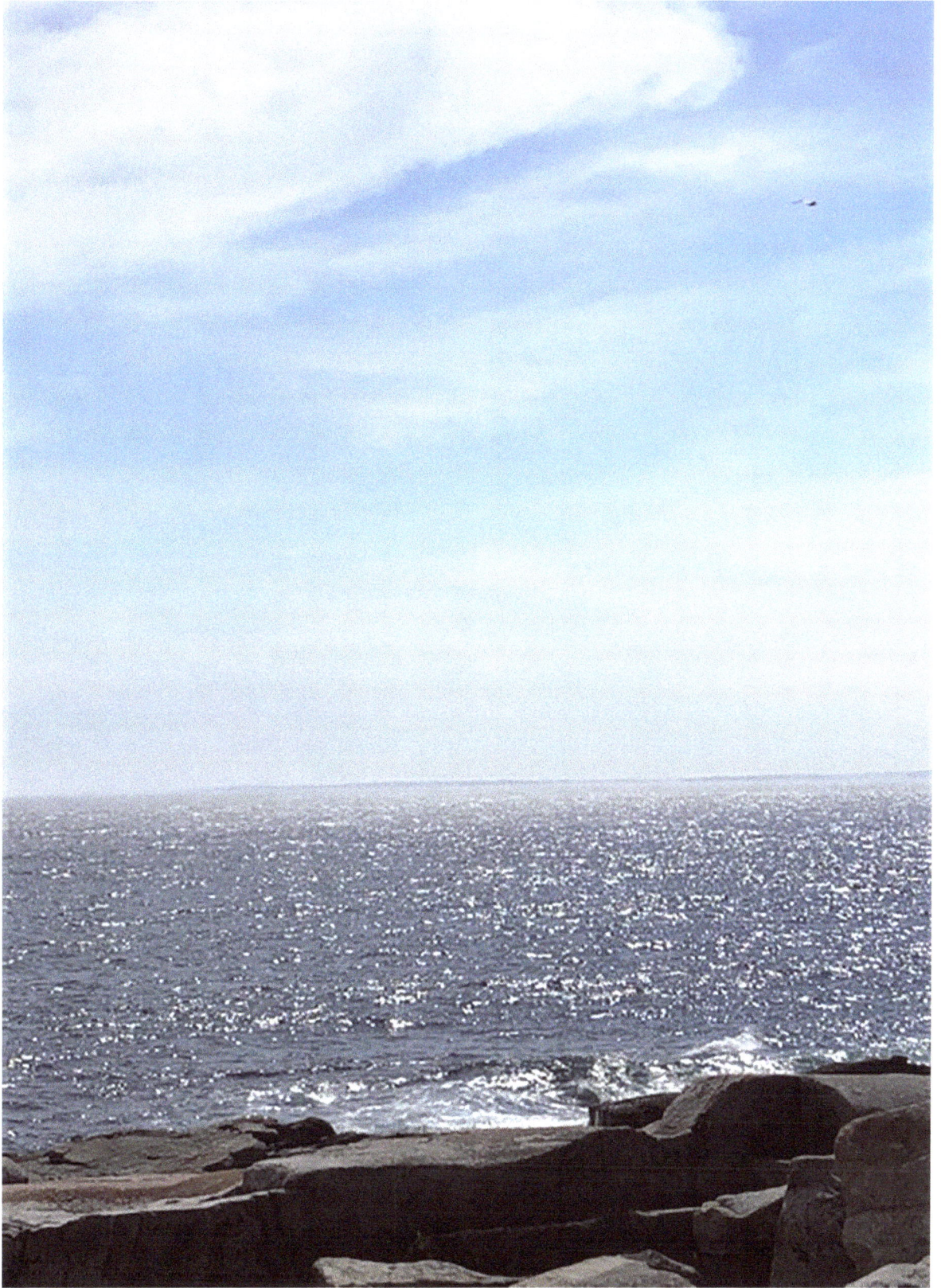

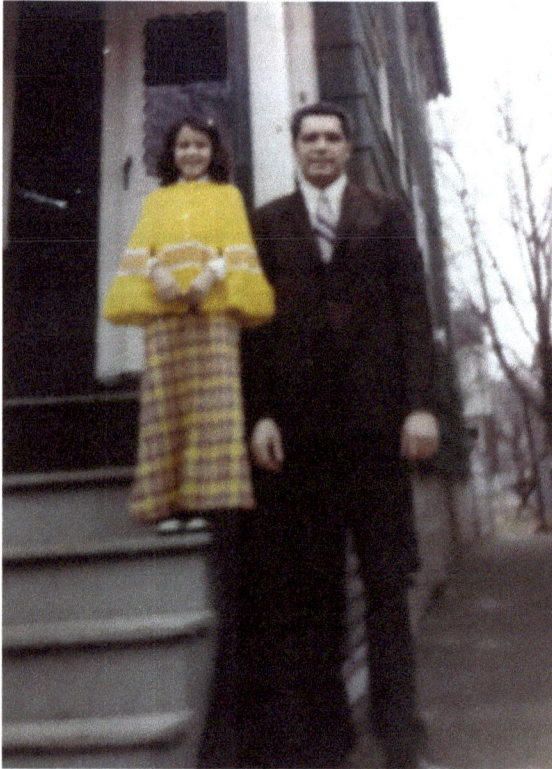

April 2020

I am sorta surprised that I love my dementia buddies. Sometimes you just don't know who is a dementia dude or not. So, I think us dementia dudes and dudettes should wear mismatching socks as a signal.

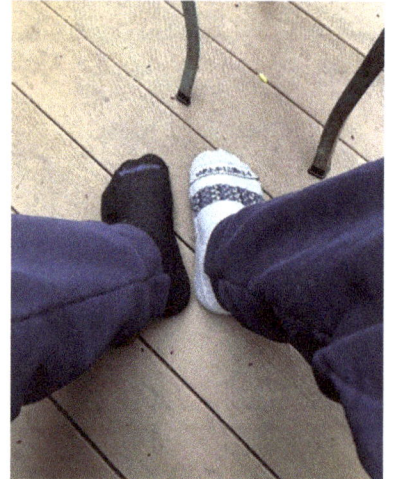

August 2, 2021

1. So I might be wrong, but dementia folks are not considered high risk. Hospitals kill us. We need to mask and so do our family and caregivers.

2. These are the worst, demeaning social ideas ever. If I had someone use this, I would leave (except if we were ordering scallops and they would give me a dementia discount).

Happy Birthday Bobo
-2021

Warm, safe and expectantly joyful
Were my early days
With a broomstick and a ball, properly mushed
Playing with my brother.

There was a rock that once was the
Foundation of the backyard that was
the scene of many a disputed call at home.
And a willow tree between the lines and
foul pole that could confound a call to the
home rock.

I am grateful to you for the extra out and
the triple header.
And sad when you victoriously went into the world.

A walkoff homerun over the fence awaits
He is holding out the hand as you round third,
tenderly and gracefully, as you did me, as we
walk barefoot in the grass, in victory again.

Love you brother.

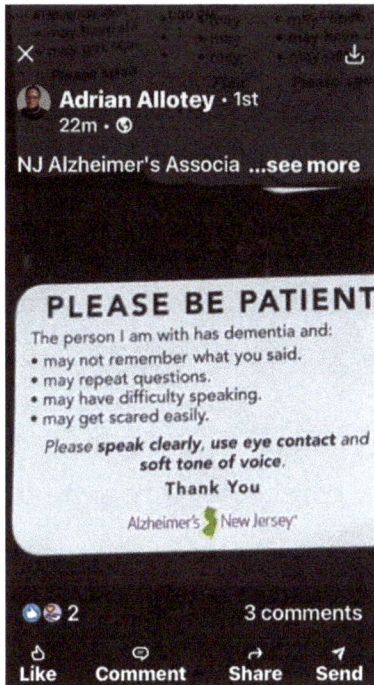

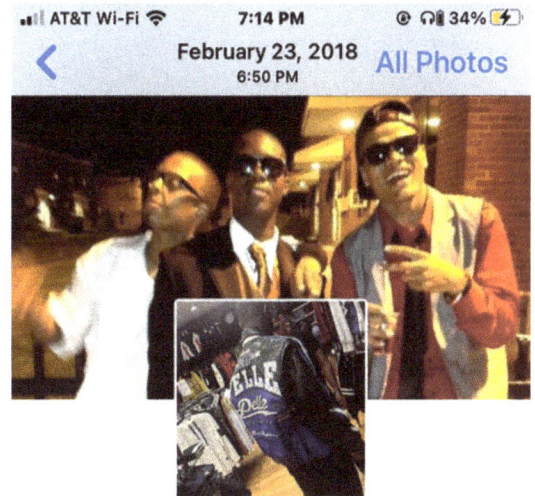

NorthTrenton Butter

I dont cut checks 💸 💵 ✉️ ..but ill pay you 💰 💵 😍 ..watchu want a stack..here take 2 😋 😉 😎

PLEASE BE PATIENT

The person I am with has dementia and:

- may not remember what you said.

- may repeat questions.

- may have difficulty speaking.

- may get scared easily.

Please speak clearly, use eye contact and a

soft tone of voice.

Thank You

Alzheimer's New Jersey

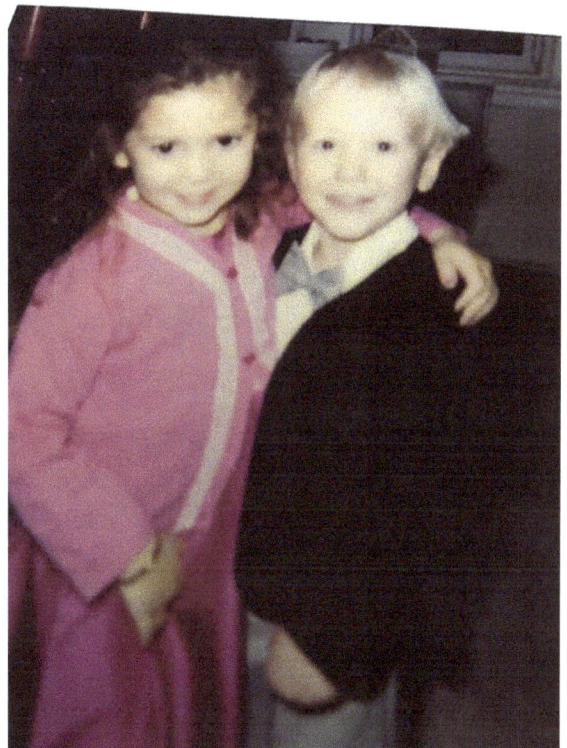

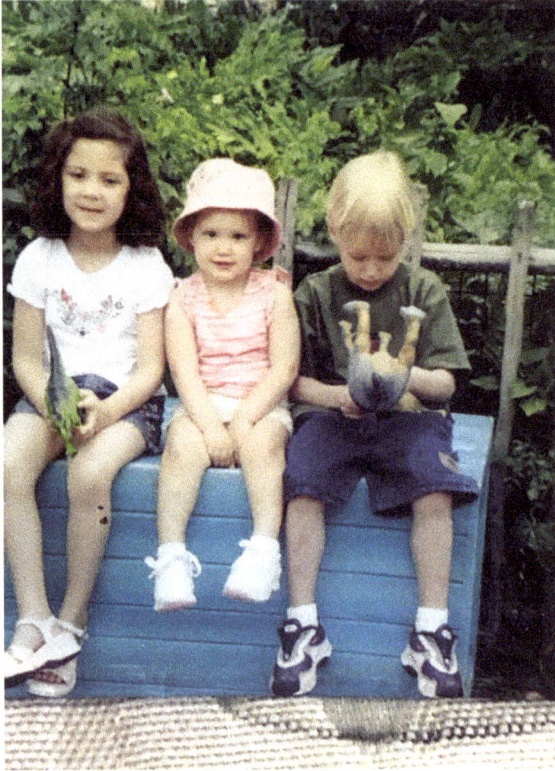

Dementia and Worship: Places of worship suck at creating dementia-friendly worship. My favorite moment was communion. I could never remember the details (a lot of them) so froze with the line of people used to "nice rushing." Thoughts? Is this the dementia or marijuana talking?

Grace and mercy should be the two most important ingredients in the reciprocal caring relationship for us dementia people and . . . all of us.

Dementia Caregivers Constitution, Article 1: All caregiving shall be reciprocal and full of grace and mercy. THE END

#HospiceWhispers #ShowingUp #PowerOfPresence #Kindness

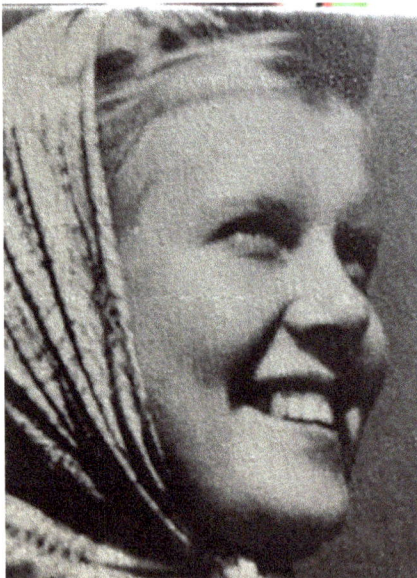

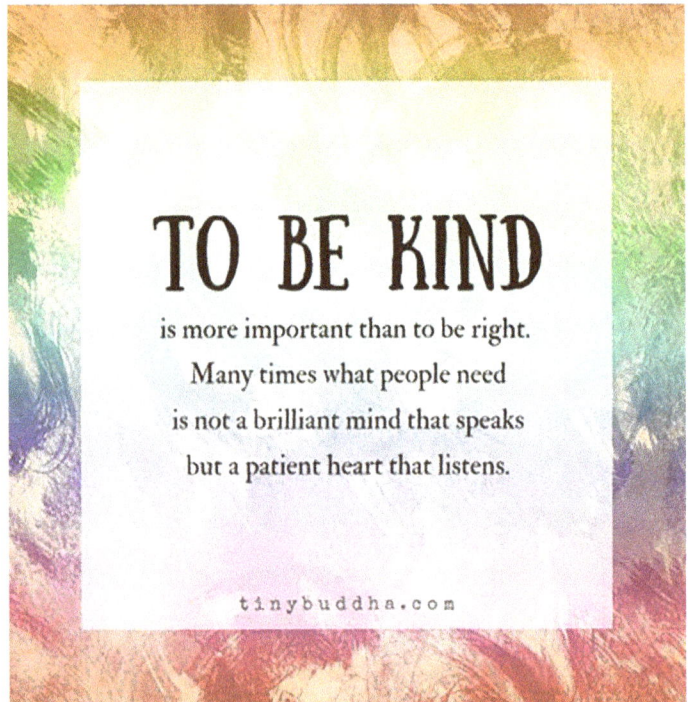

TO BE KIND
is more important than to be right.
Many times what people need
is not a brilliant mind that speaks
but a patient heart that listens.

tinybuddha.com

👍❤️🫂 11   3 comments

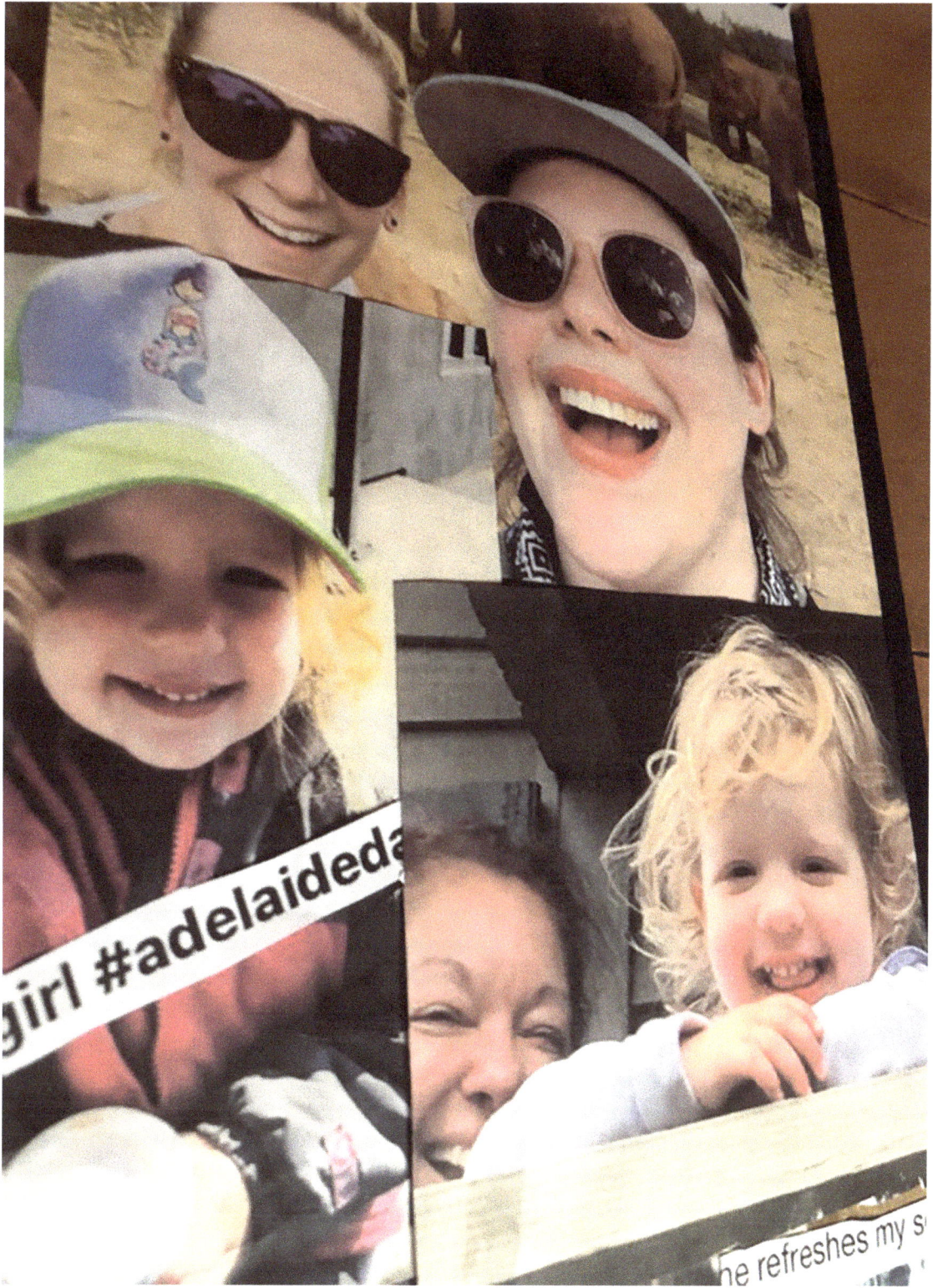

girl #adelaideda

he refreshes my s

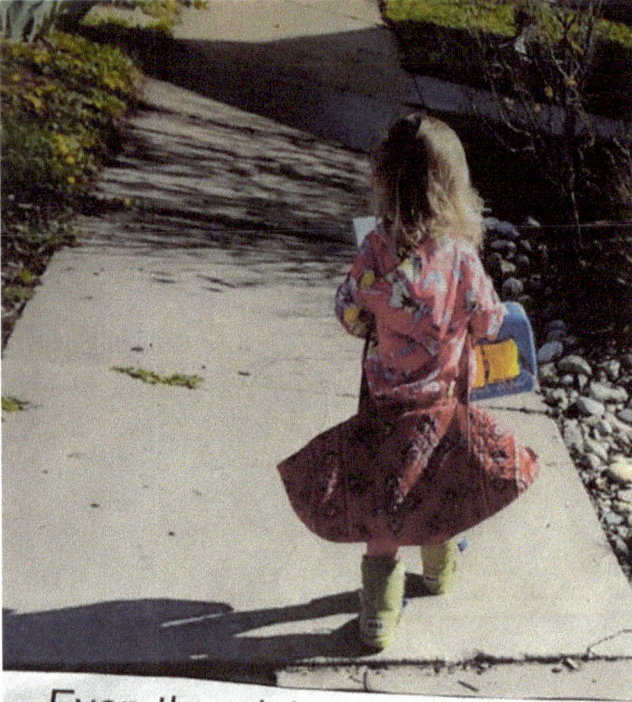

Even though I walk
through the darkest valley,[a]
I will fear no evil,
for you are with me;

Am I out of line feeling as if dementia folks are being used once again? Should we be embarrassed to ask about side effects? And if it doesn't affect cognitive decline, what does it do? Alzheimer's Association should be ashamed at raising expectations, while raising dollars by casting us as veggies. Resign, Harry. It's a new day. We have learned to not wait around for the scraps off your association table. Harry, tell me it is not true that you make a million dollars salary.

Even though I walk

through the darkest valley,

I will fear no evil,

for you are with me...

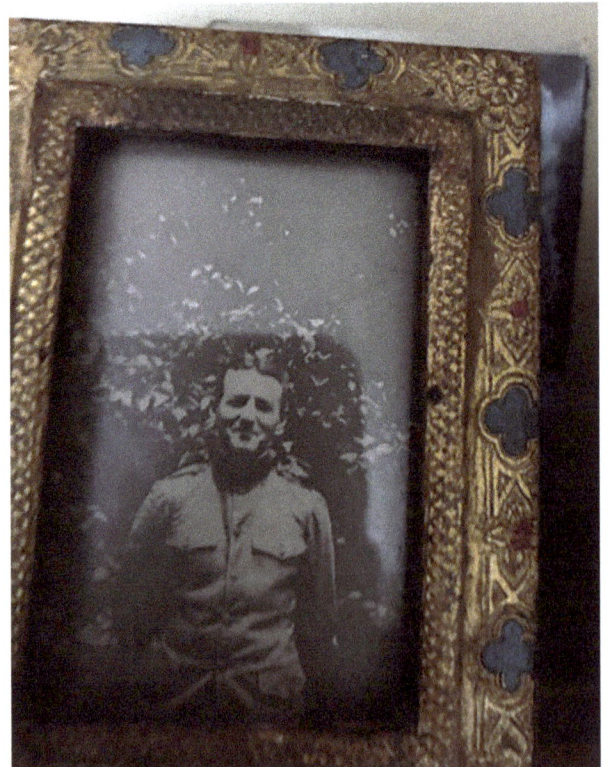

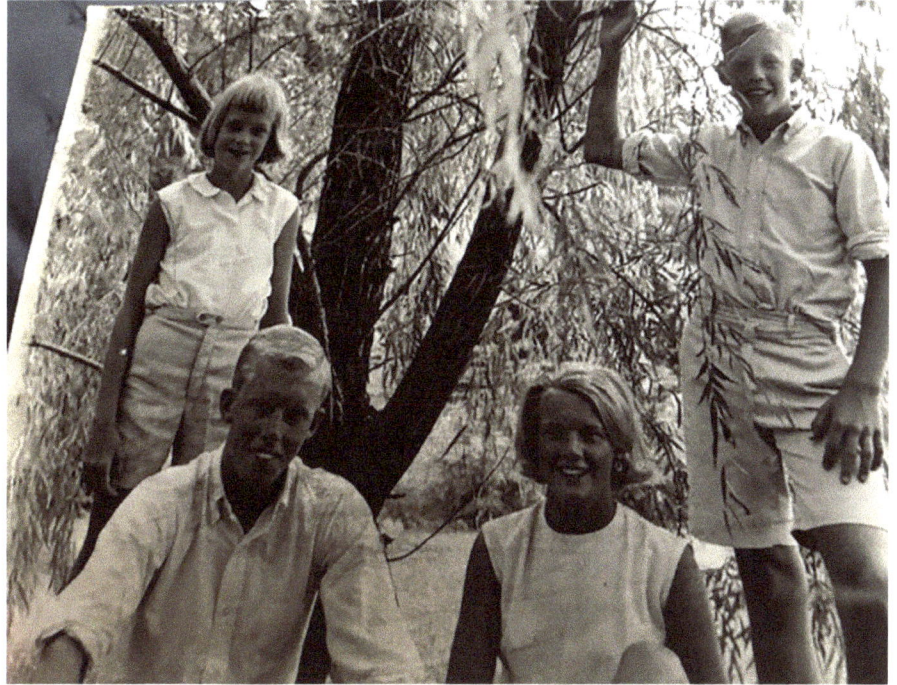

Three F.D.A. Advisers Resign Over Agency's Approval of Alzheimer's Drug

The drug, Aduhelm, a monthly infusion priced at $56,000 per year, was approved this week despite weak evidence

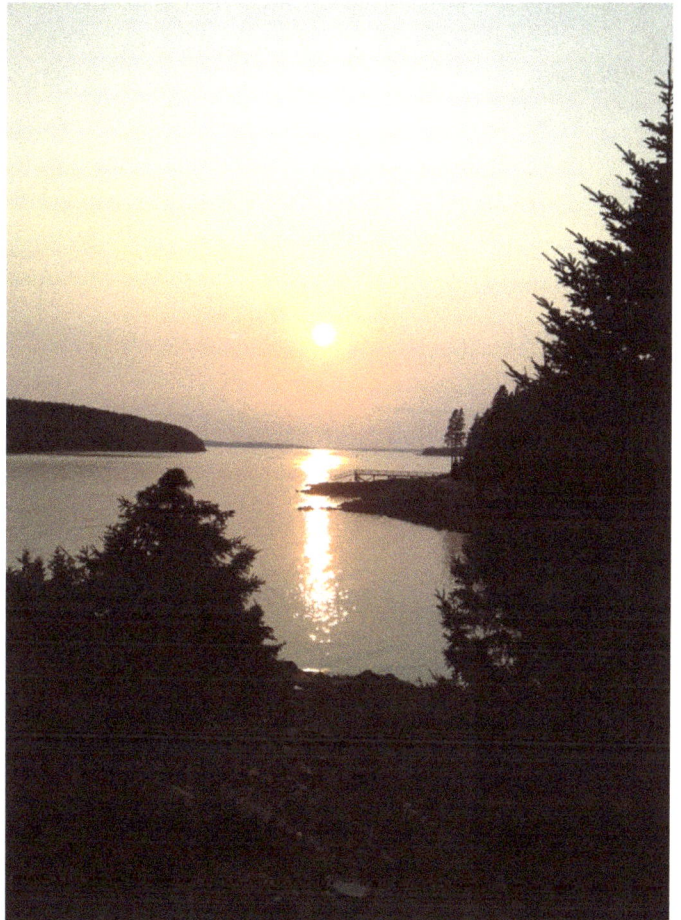

April 2020

COVID-19 and dementia. The good thing is that we have had years of practicing to be ready to die. Ahead of the game. Isolation? We have grown used to this too. Not knowing who or what to believe? No problem, this is dementia 101.

July 2020

I am officially declaring the inability of planning . . . pretty much anything. Apologies to regular people, but for us this is great news. Happy July 4, dementia dudes and dudettes. Dementia is getting better and better.

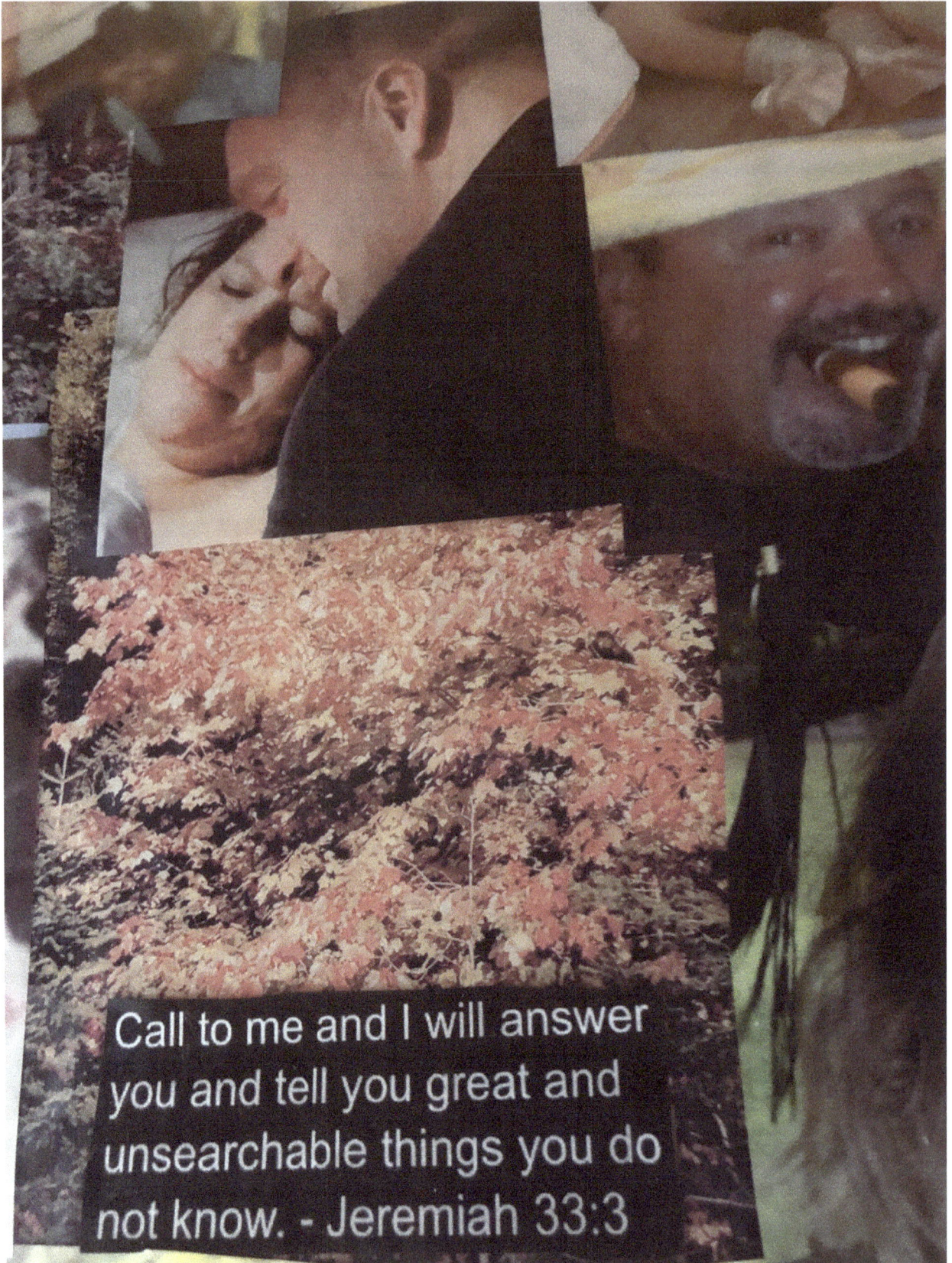

Call to me and I will answer you and tell you great and unsearchable things you do not know. - Jeremiah 33:3

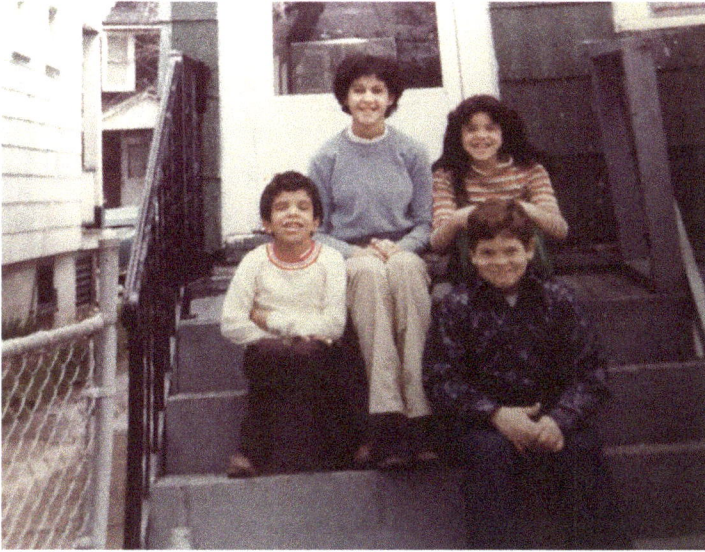

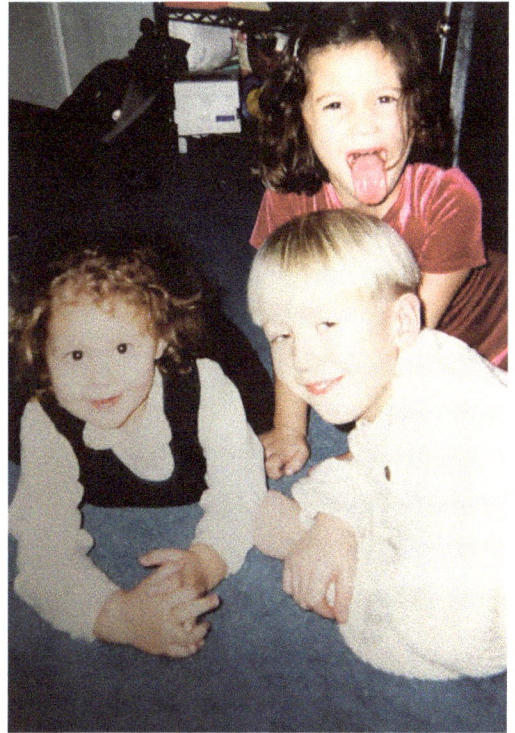

For us dementia people or the pros: So COVID creates brain fog. Dementia creates brain fog. So does that equal 2 brain fogs? If so our cognition and or living environment is hit with lightening . And furthermore this fact makes all dementia folks high risk. . .

Are we so chacterized? Should we ? Ironic right? The organizations play up our doomsday credentials for their benefit? And now ?

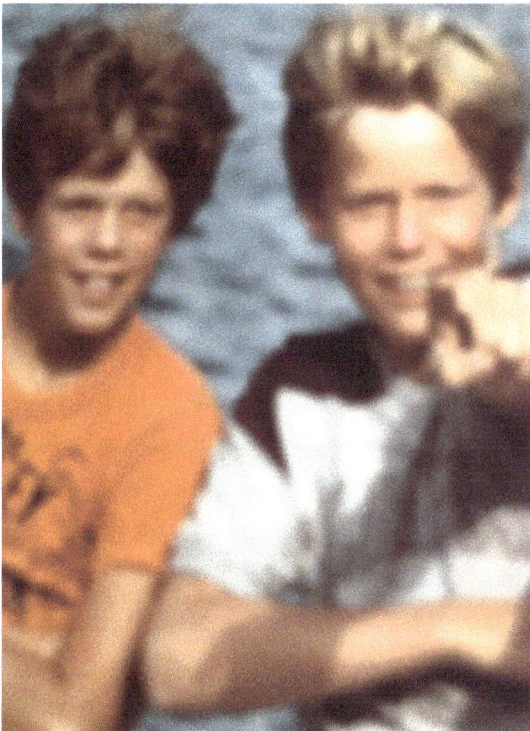

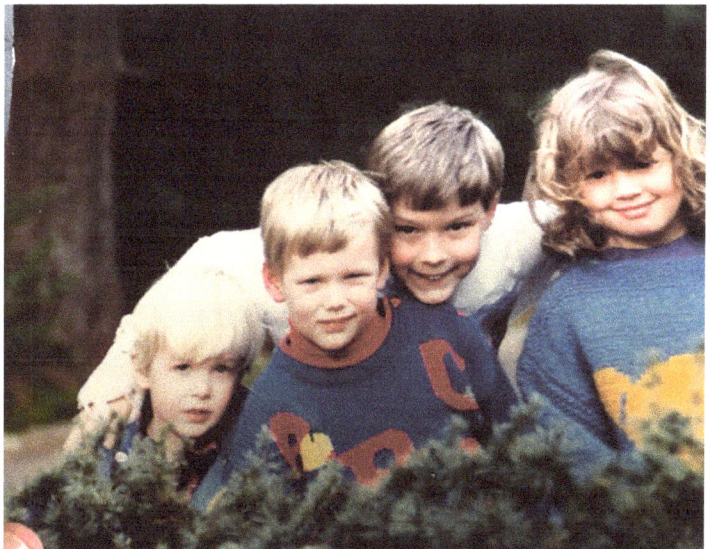

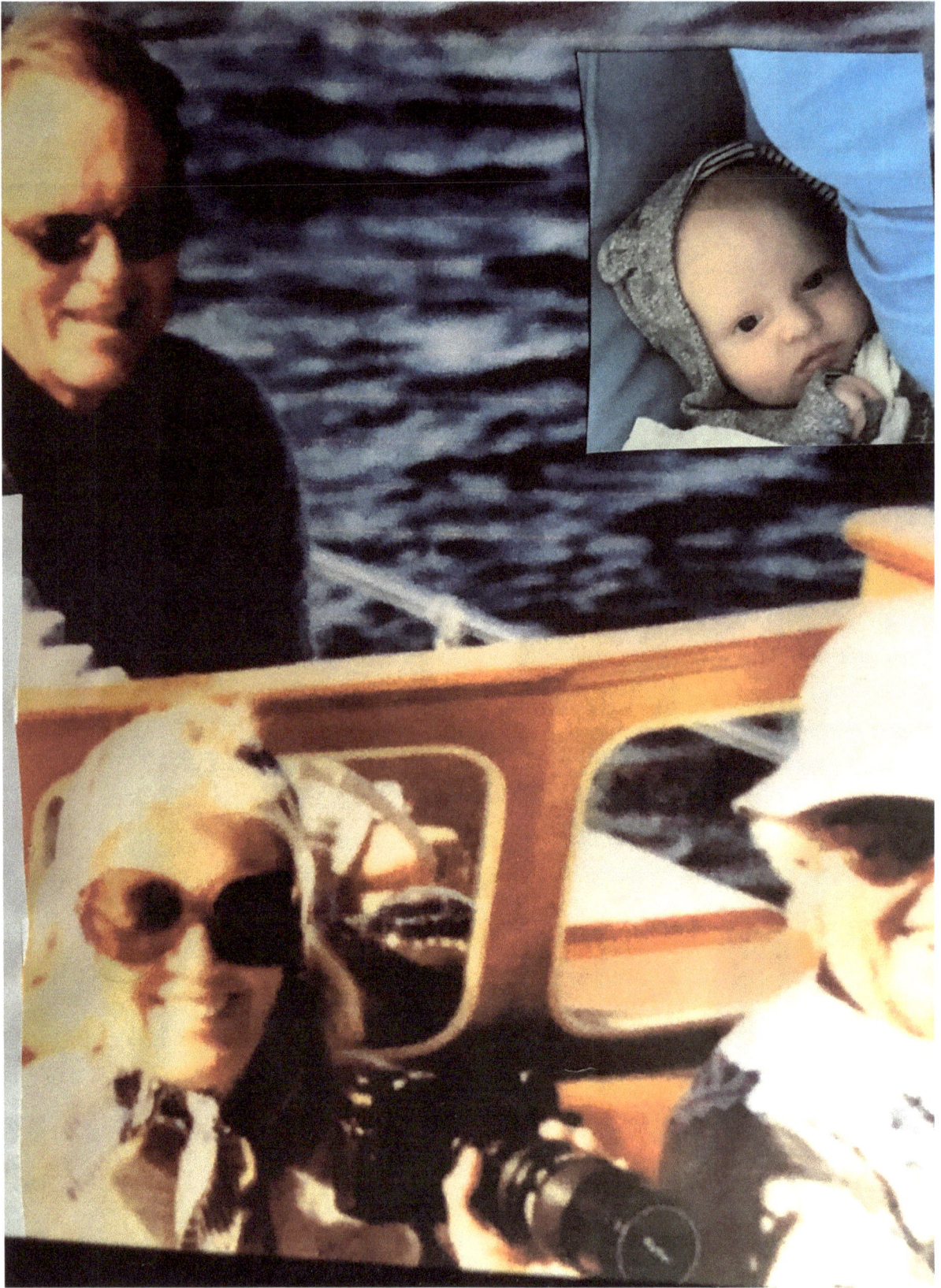

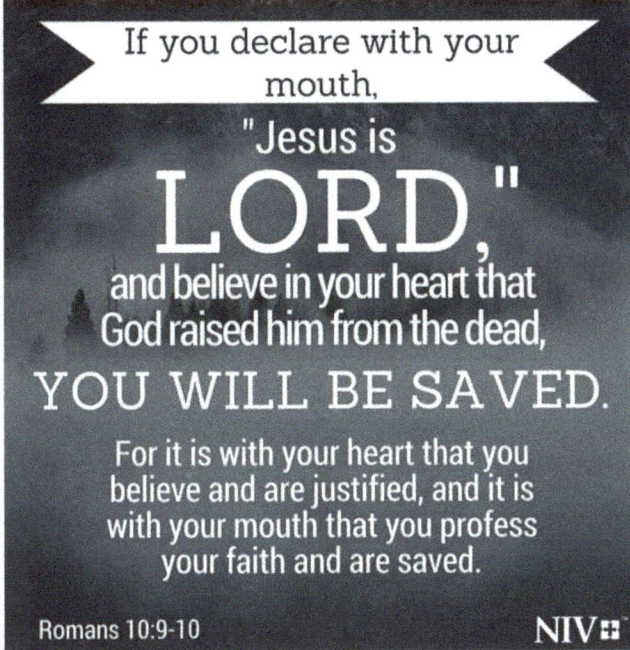

mekala Prakash • 1st
Servant of God at calvary blood of Christ ministries
52m • 🌐

I pray for all my family and friends to come to the saving knowledge of Jesus Christ.

If you declare with your mouth,
"Jesus is
LORD,"
and believe in your heart that God raised him from the dead,
YOU WILL BE SAVED.
For it is with your heart that you believe and are justified, and it is with your mouth that you profess your faith and are saved.
Romans 10:9-10   NIV

👍 Like   💬 Comment   ↗ Share   ✈ Send

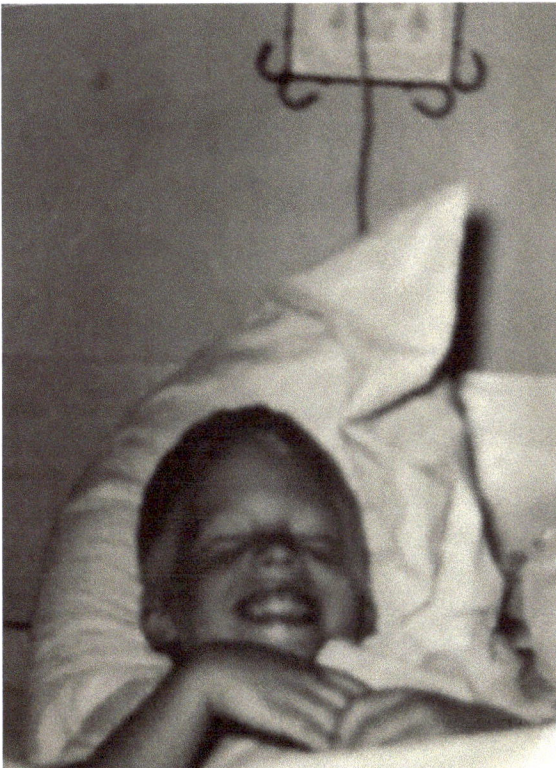

Let My He...   Done
David & Nicole Bini...

Can't find the words to express what I'm feeling inside

Every time I see your face

I get lost in your eyes

You sing a love song of heaven and my heart starts to cry

Shadows of pain are eclipsed by Your healing light

My deep sorrow erased by Your love so bright

You stroll my heart with your Song

And I feel so alive, I feel so alive

21

Let My He...　　Done

David & Nicole Bini...

You gave me beauty for ashes

You changed my sorrow to joy

You turned my mourning to dancing

So I'll let my heart dance

I'm overwhelmed by You

As I began to love myself
I quit trying to always be right,
and ever since I was wrong less of
the time.

Today I discovered that is Modesty.

As I began to love myself
I refused to go on living in the past
and worrying about the future.
Now, I only live for the moment,
where everything is happening.

Today I live each day, day by day,
and I call it Fulfillment.

As I began to love myself
I recognized that my mind can
disturb me
and it can make me sick.
But as I connected it to my heart,
my mind became a valuable ally.

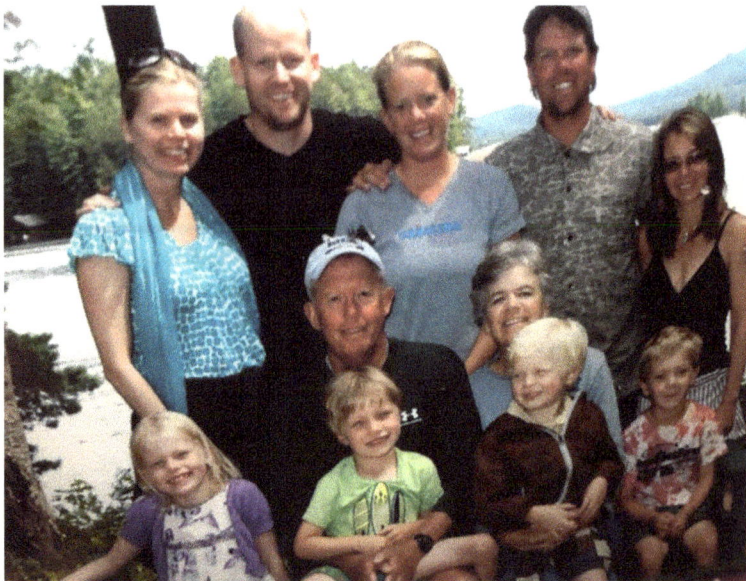

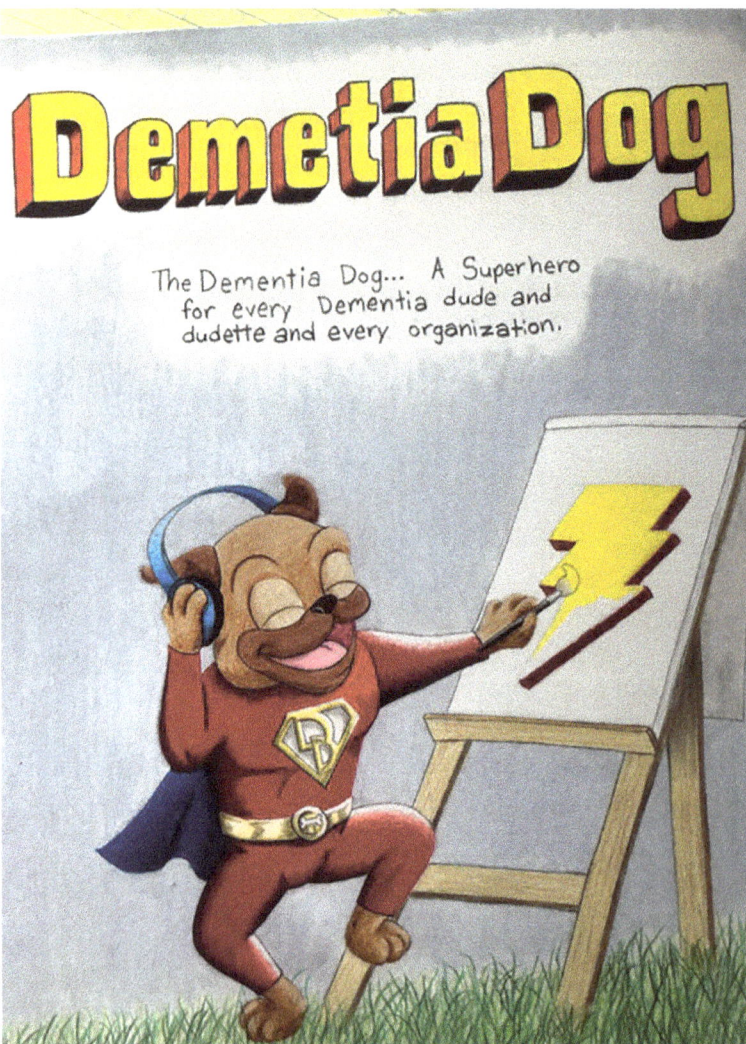

DemetiaDog

The Dementia Dog... A Superhero
for every Dementia dude and
dudette and every organization.

by Emil Fennel

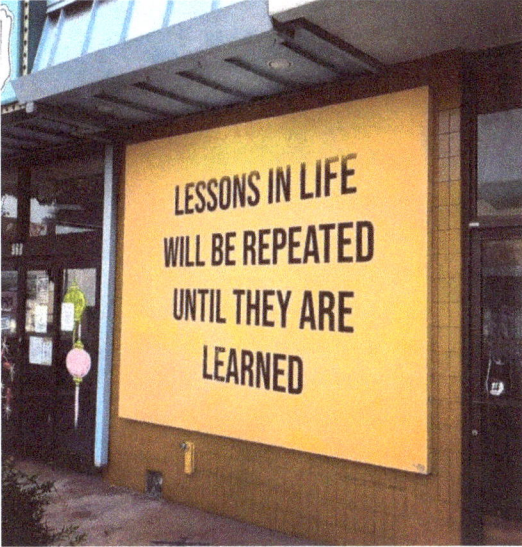

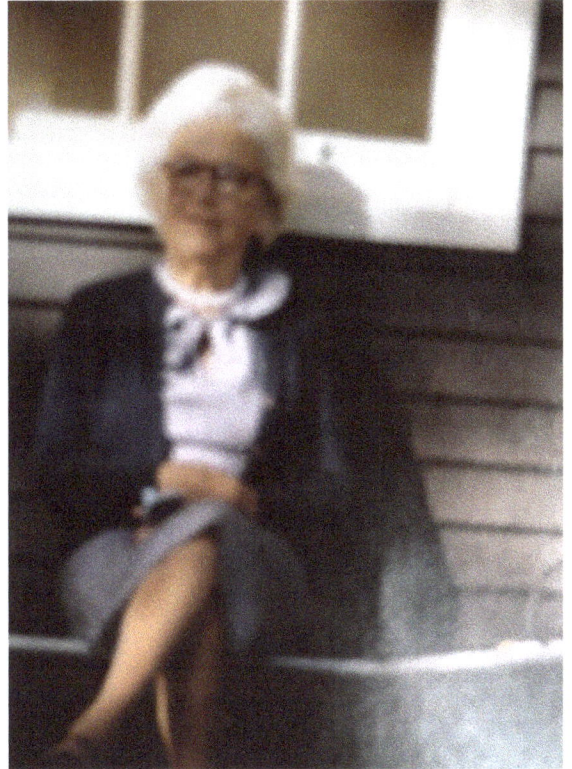

"I'm so much more than my dementia, as is everybody."

Bobby Redman,
Dementia advocate

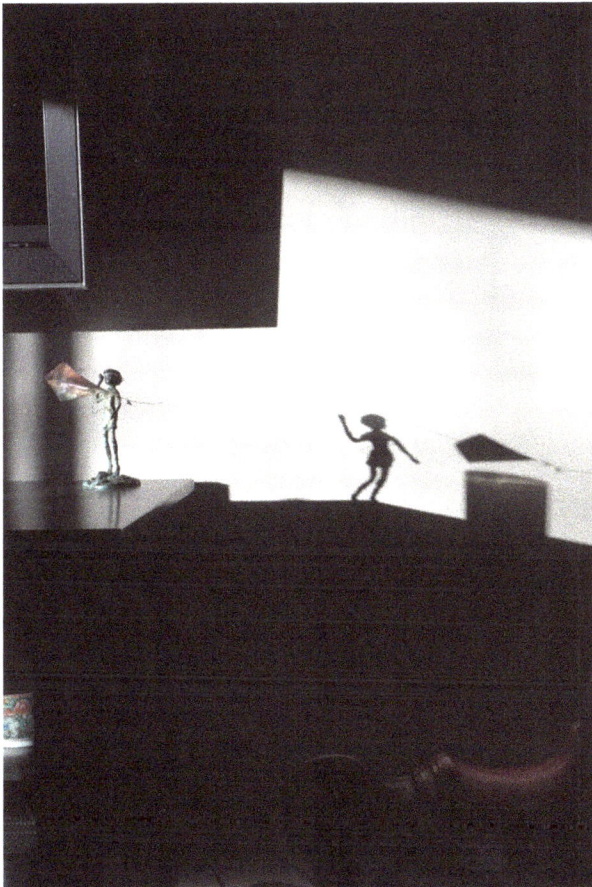

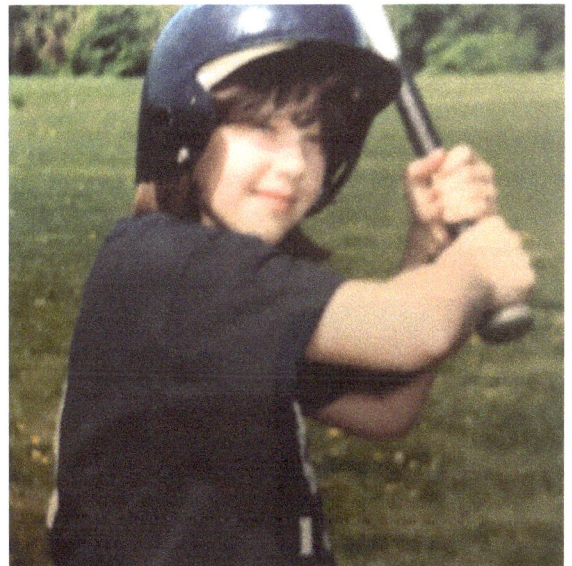

Warning: The most dangerous part of dementia and forgetting you have it. Why? Because others take control and they usually know way less than we do. And out of the good routine we developed over lots of trial and error that we can't reconstruct.

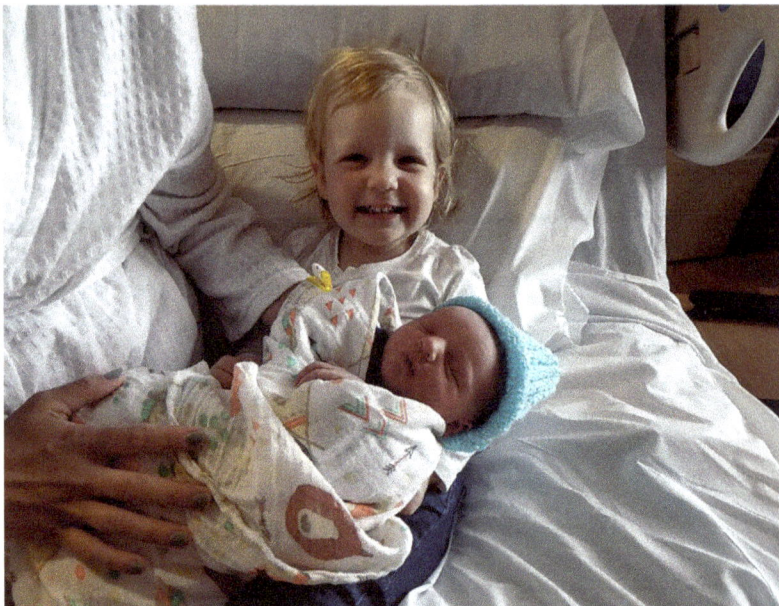

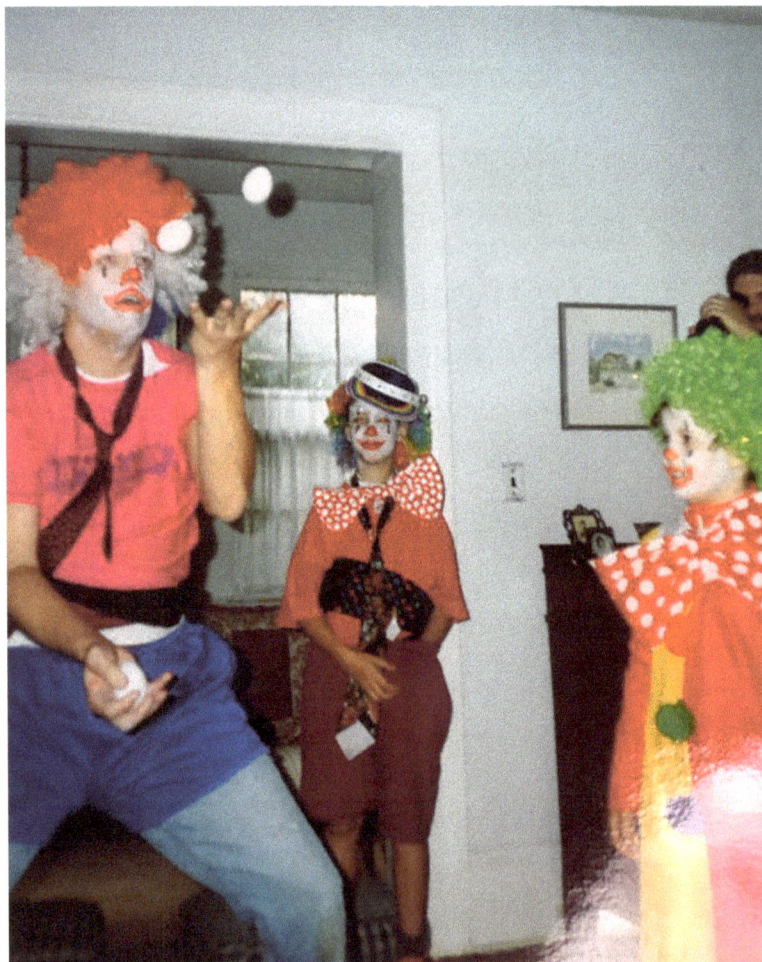

March 2021

I now know this is simplistic even for us dementia people, but for seven years I couldn't figure out why it seemed I was busy, when in reality I wasn't doing much at all. I missed the fact that it takes me twice as long (and perhaps twice the effort). Time bending.

March 2021

Can we skip one bingo game (where the prizes usually suck) and instead conduct a class to teach us how to die? Us is old dementia people who are usually uninvited to the class, even if there is one.

November 2020

I'm sureish I'm not the first to say that the simple difference between a faulty memory (age related or not) and us having a dementiafried memory is that it does us no good to search for the lost item or thought. Oh, you might find it sometimes, but it's rarely worth the effort.

November 2020

Dementia itself doesn't cause fear; our reaction to it does. My dad used to lament that Alzheimer's was the worst possible thing to happen to somebody. Someone screwed up our public relations early, early.

Constance Kelley
1 hr · 🌐

The Dementia Declaration of Independence

We, the people living with dementia, our friends, family, caregivers, and supporters, no longer accept the dying vegetable label. Nor do we condone the use of this and other false narratives by organizations for their purposes.

We declare that folks with dementia have a super power that protects certain joys from cognitive decline: music appreciation, the delight of play, deep love, spiritual memory, a sense of humor, the ability to read tones of voice, and numerous and various artistic expressions, which include painting, poetry, woodworking, gardening, dance, bird watching, and many others.

We declare these joys to be self-evident. They are our right in our pursuit of happiness, joy, and safety. It is our personal and corporate expectation whatever setting we are in.

From the Dementia Dudes and Dudettes at Dementia Action International

**"Let us fight as if it all depended upon us, but let us look up and know that all depends upon HIM (GOD)."
Charles Spurgeon**

Dallas Dixon likes this   ...

Denise T. · 2nd
Ex-HR Pro | EAP Counsellor | Guidance Counsellor
3w · 🌐

"He is 85 and insists on taking his wife's hand everywhere they go. When I asked him why his wife kept looking away, he responded, 'because she has Alzheimer's.' I then proceeded to ask him, 'will your wife worry if yc ...see more

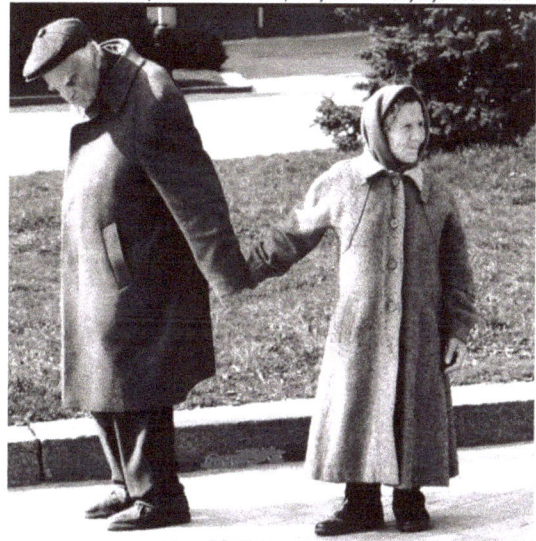

👍❤️ 15   3 Comments

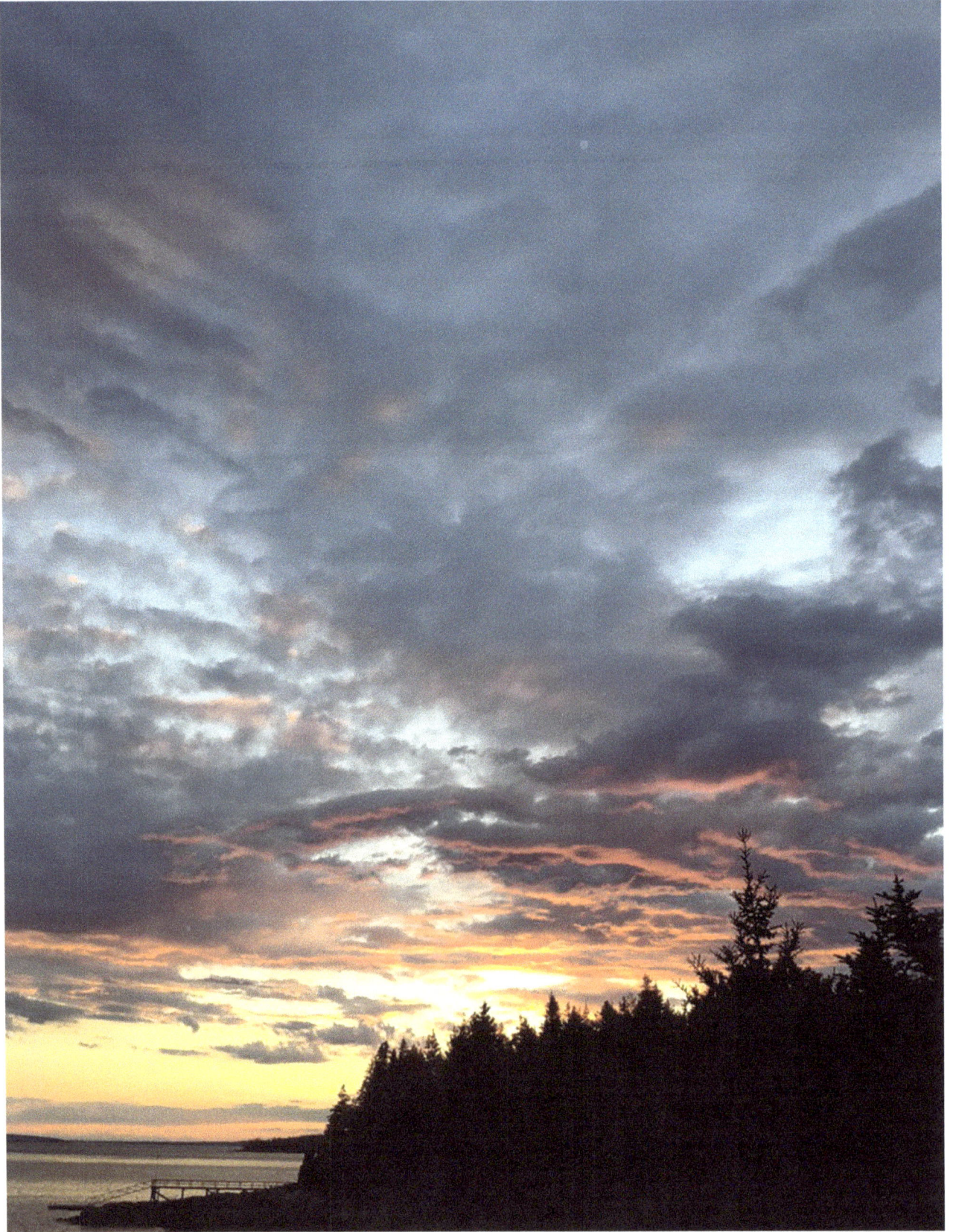

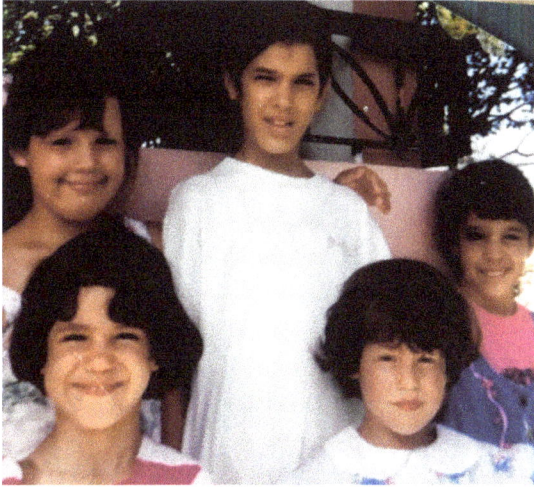

Be completely humble and gentle;
be patient, bearing with one another
in love.

Ephesians 4:2

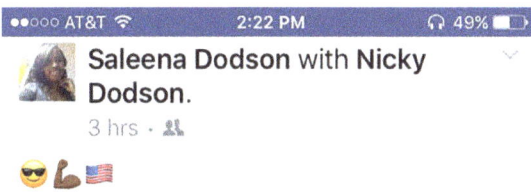

●●○○○ AT&T 📶   2:22 PM   🎧 49% 🔋

Saleena Dodson with **Nicky Dodson**.

3 hrs · 👥

😎 💪🏾 🇺🇸

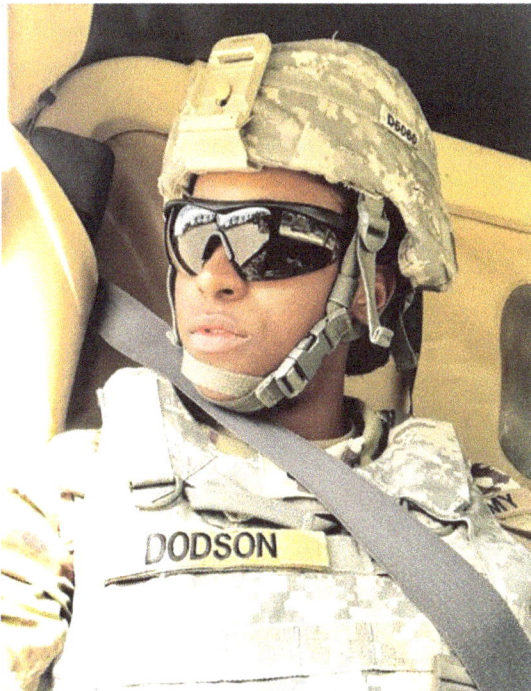

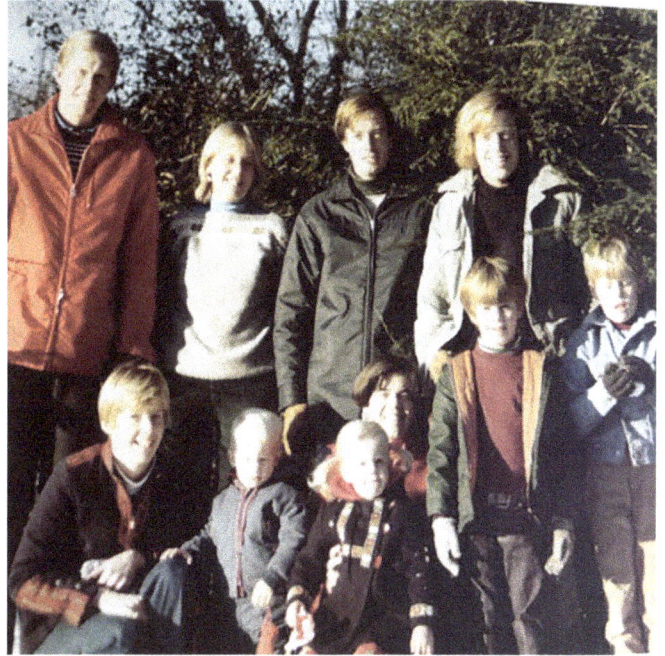

September 2020
Dementia folks have abundant
opportunities to show amazing grace,
tender mercies, and loving kindnesses.
Maybe that's just our new job.

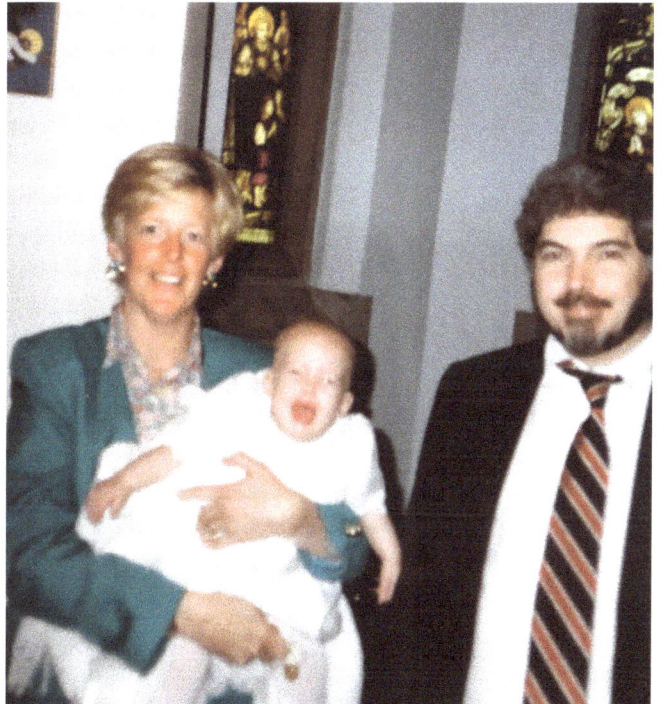

Warning to regulars and us dementia people. Don't interfere with God's miracles. Why would we except that we think we can do better? I'm pretty sure I'm right about this after trying it.

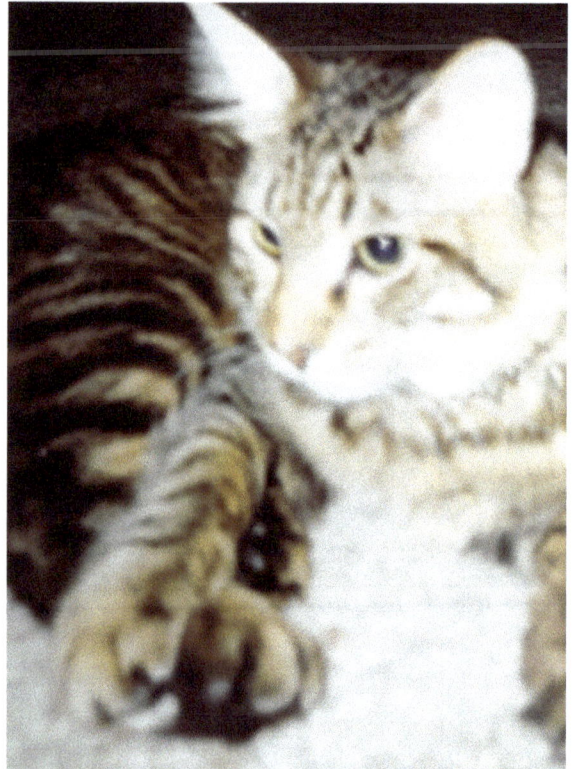

●●○○○ AT&T LTE   8:48 AM   ✳ 76% ▬

Great Is Your...   Done
Donnie McClurkin — Th...

Your loving kindness toward me

Your tender mercies I see

Day after day

Forever faithful to me

Always providing for me

Great is Your mercy toward me

Great is Your grace

Your promises are ageless

Your Love will never end

To a thousand generations

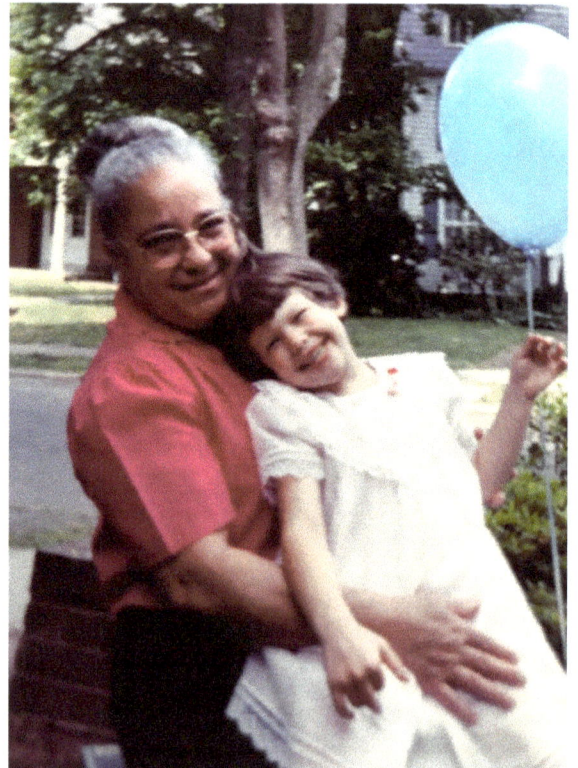

Standing (Live)　　Done
William McDowell & Mar...

Can you hear the voice of the Father

Inviting you to walk the water?

Risk it all, answer the call, and enter in.

Now we stand on every promise

We're not afraid, our faith goes before us

When we believe, we're gonna see

The supernatural

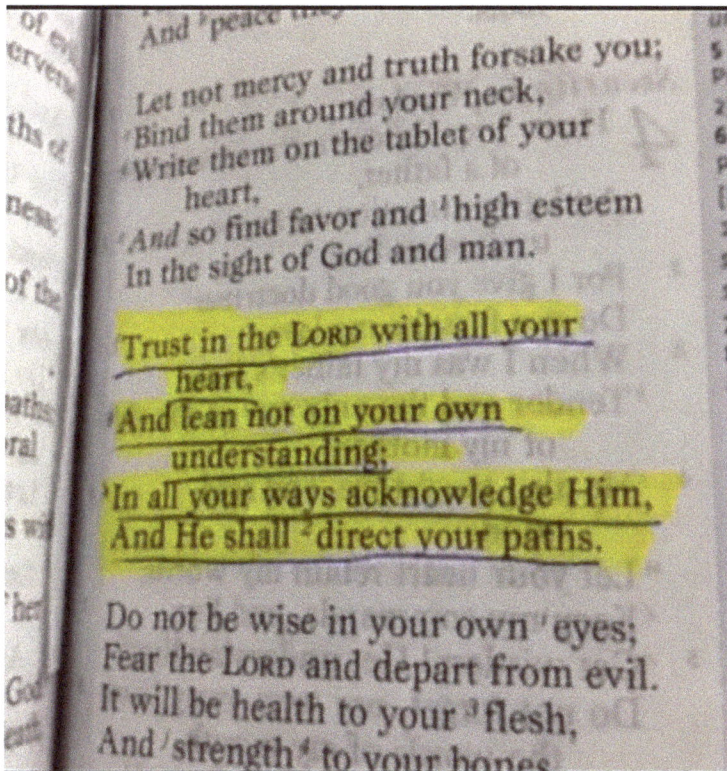

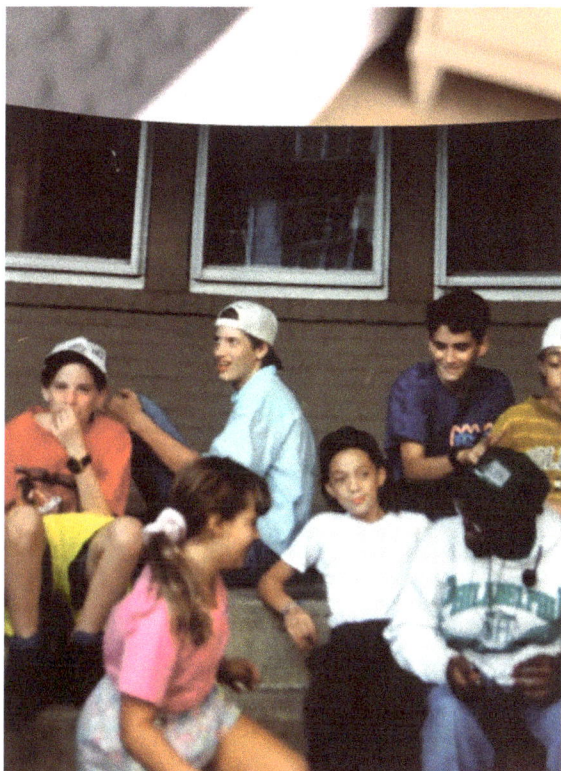

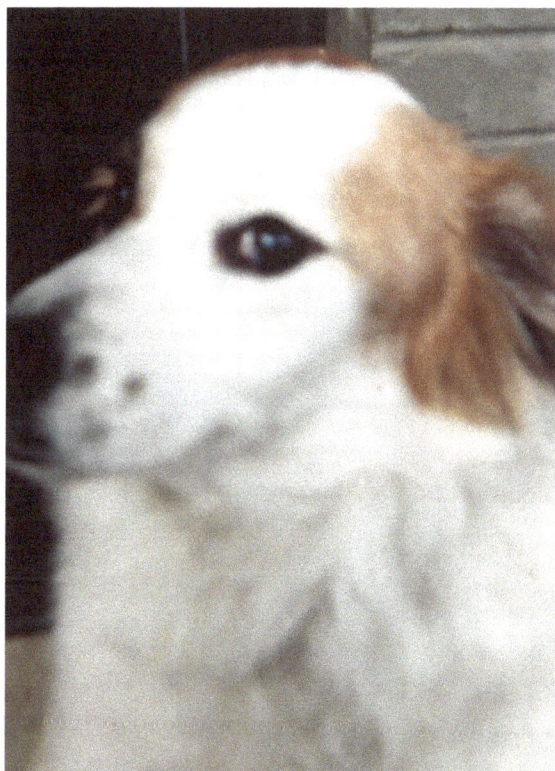

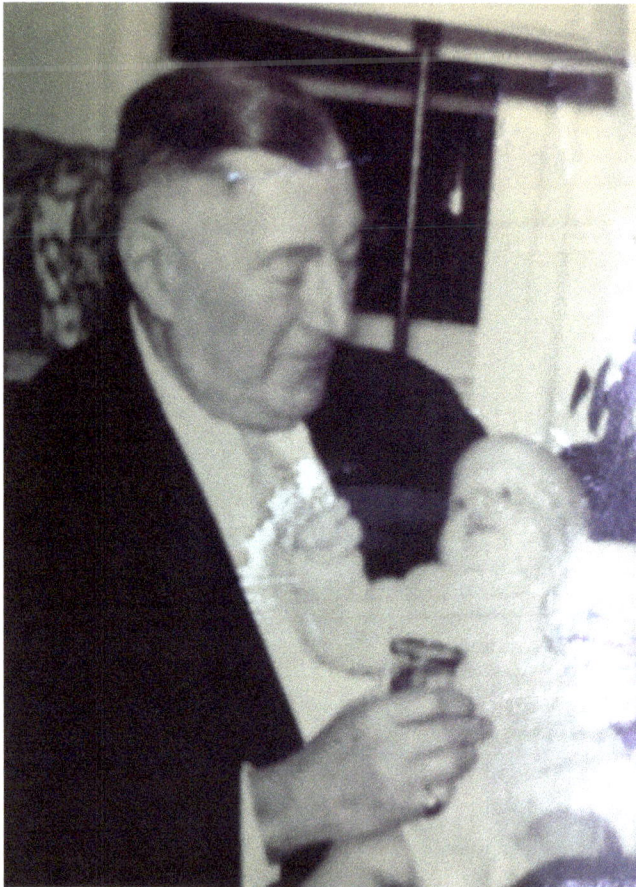

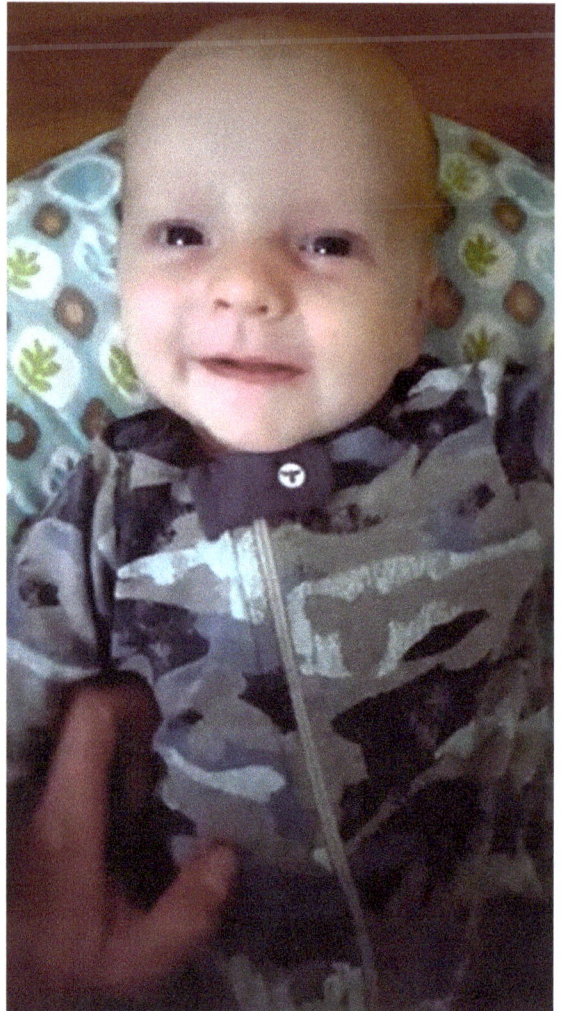

So this dementia dude been pondering. If you've been around the dementia world some, you all well-acquainted with regular people saying, "You don't look like you have dementia," which is calling us a mentally ill fraud. Not nice on this end.

So I told a family member how I thought it was dementia funny when I get lost in my sweater /hoodie while putting it on. Reply: "Oh that happens to everybody." Soft version of the above. Not pleasant. But in this case, it is conceivably true. But you regular folks give the passive aggressive away. We can still read your disdainful superior tone of voice.

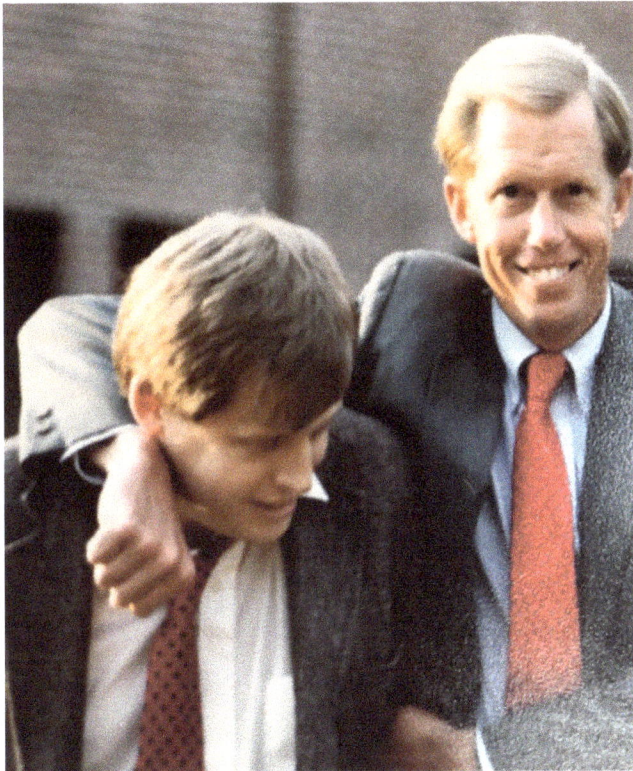

Love is patient, love is kind. It does not envy, it does not boast, it is not proud. It does not dishonor others, it is not self-seeking, it is not easily angered, it keeps no record of wrongs.

I Corinthians 13:4-5

●●○○○ AT&T 📶　　　6:56 PM　　　◌ 🎧 63% 🔋

I Know the Pl...　　Done
Martha Munizzi — The...

So when you can't see
What tomorrow holds
And yesterday is through,
Remember I know,
The plans I have for you

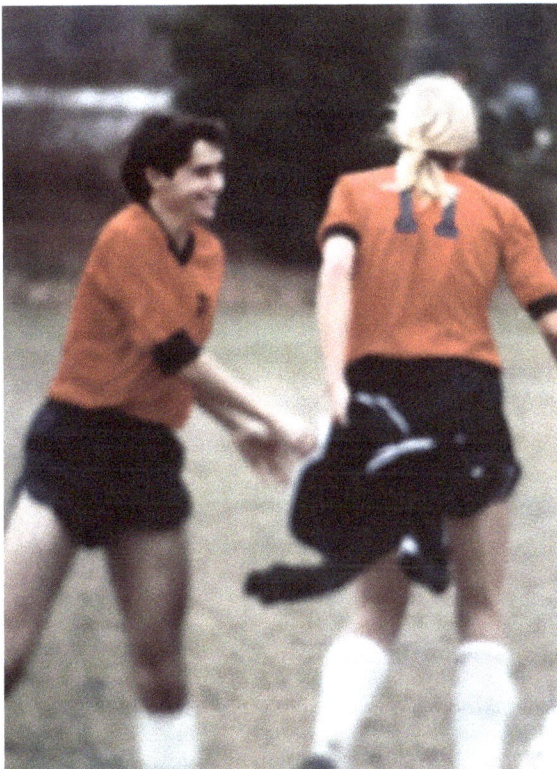

To give you hope for tomorrow
Joy for your sorrow
Strength for everything you go through
Remember I know the plans I have for you

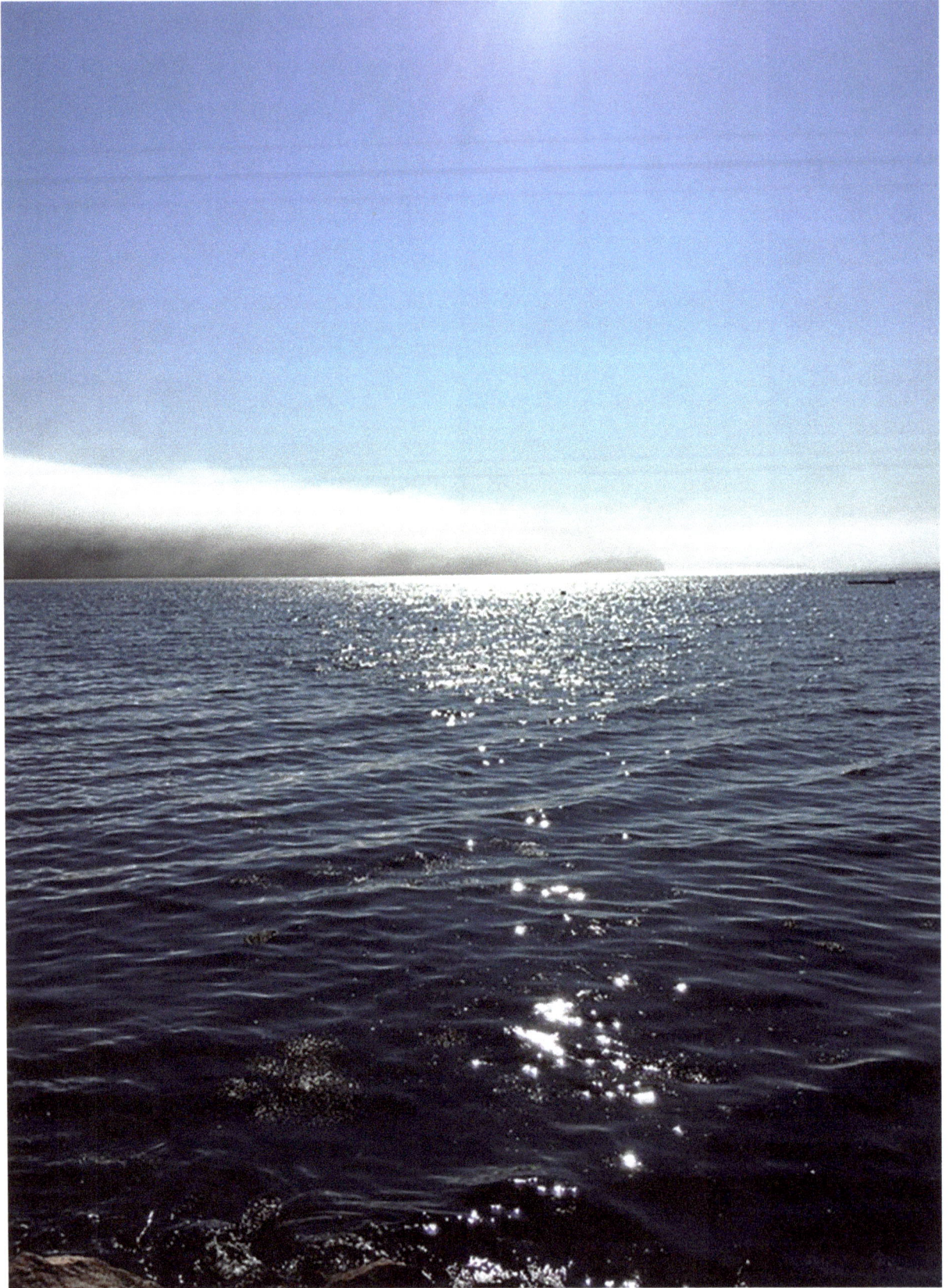

Sometimes,
when I say
"Im okay."
I want someone
to look me in
the eyes, hug me
tight and say,
"I know you're
not."

via curiano.com

Sunday, July 16

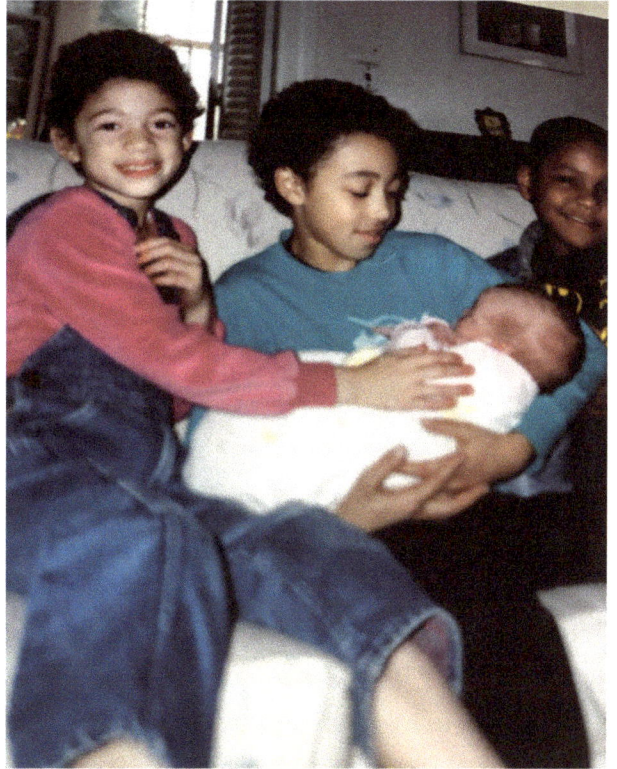

Do everything in love.

I Corinthians 16:14

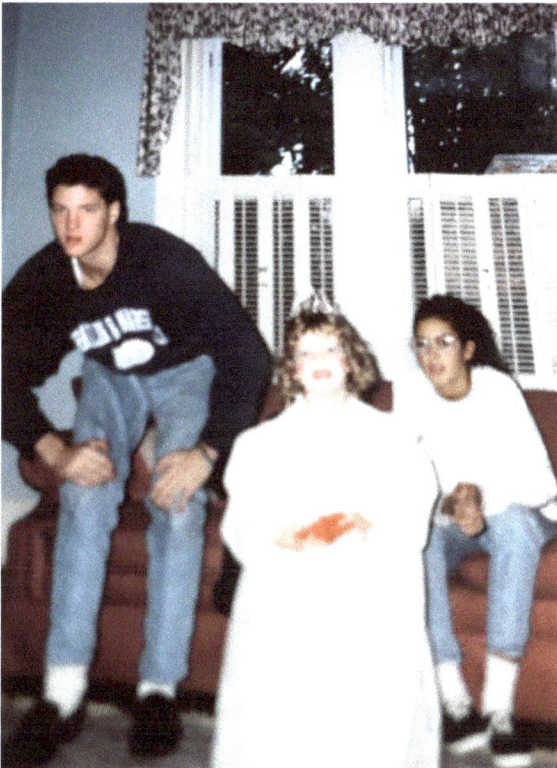

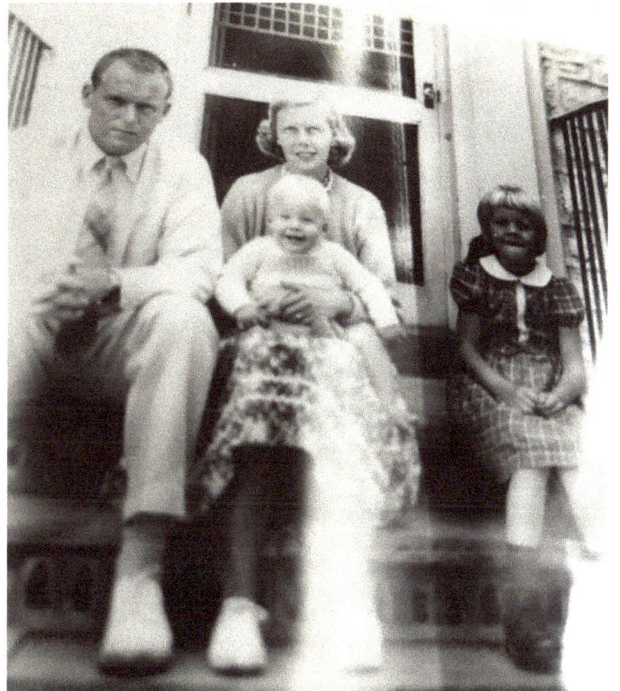

#SundayFunday

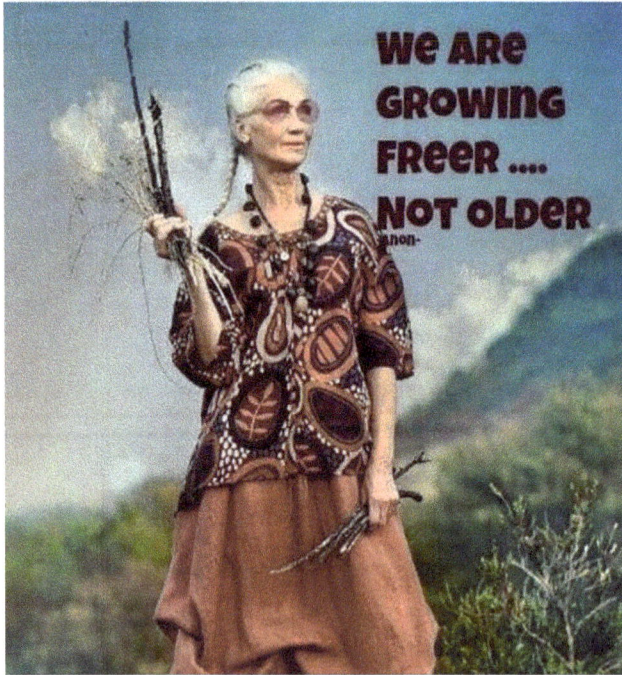

WE ARE GROWING FREER .... NOT OLDER
-anon-

HEADLINE: THREE F.D.A. ADVISERS RESIGN OVER AGENCY'S APPROVAL OF ALZHEIMER'S DRUG
The drug, Aduhelm, a monthly infusion priced at $56,000 per year, was approved this week despite weak evidence.

Many dementia folks' hopes have gone through the roof with the news of this new "drug" Aduhelm. Shame on the corporate folks, who failed to warn, and the dementia community, who applauded the deception (again). Alzheimer's leaders who went along blindfolded for the ride should confess or resign.

Dementia can be counterintuitive. I'm busy. My sleep and memory issues make the days shorter along with my inability to figure what I should do first and which metro to use to decide. FYI.

Forgetting is funny a bunch of the time. Dementia Hall of Fame will most certainly have penultimate forgetters. Nominations are open. We won't let you shame us into hiding from "this is your third time asking."

Ms Louise from Swan Island said it best: "It's not the stuff you forget that's the problem; it's the stuff you can't forget that is harder to deal with."

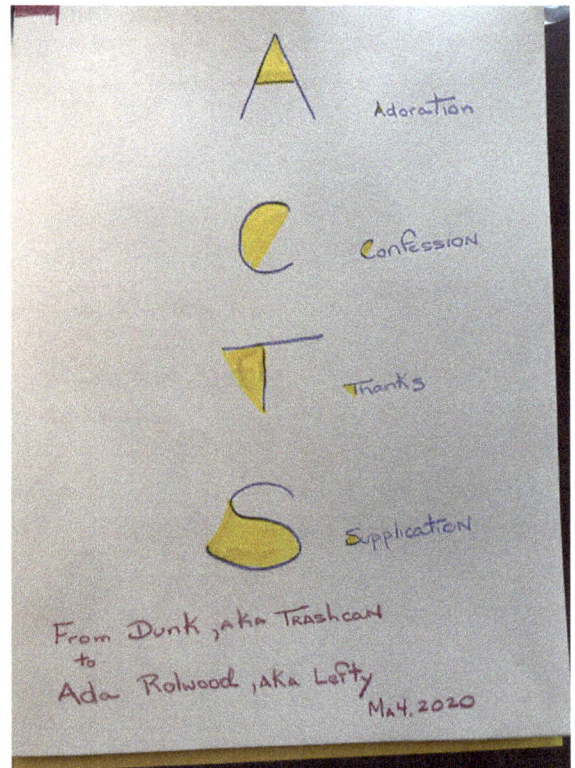

A — Adoration
C — Confession
T — Thanks
S — Supplication

From Dunk, aka Trashcan
to
Ada Rolwood, aka Lefty
May 2020

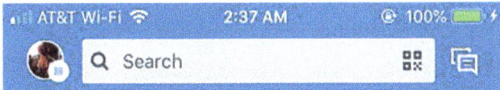
Write a post

Amen! 😭🙏😊

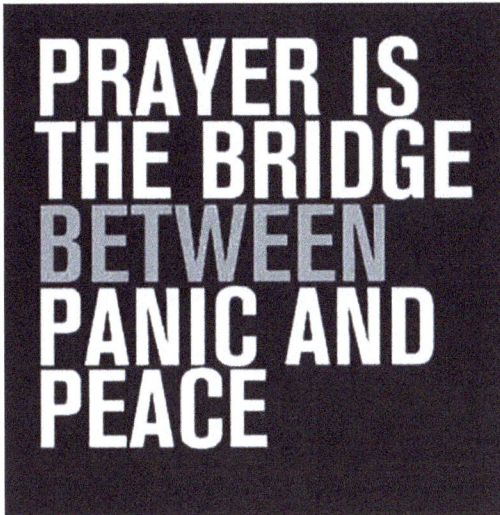

PRAYER IS THE BRIDGE BETWEEN PANIC AND PEACE

18   5 Comments

Dementia Tidbit: Sometimes dementia folks are correct about something. I admit that's far less than we think (that we are on the money). But when we are, the fact that we have dementia makes it improbable that we prevail. I've held a grudge about how unfair and convoluted that truth was and the difficulty and energy sapping it would be changing it. God gave me the answer last night and again this a.m. "Do all things without complaining and disputing." Giggle . . . I used to be a criminal trial attorney.

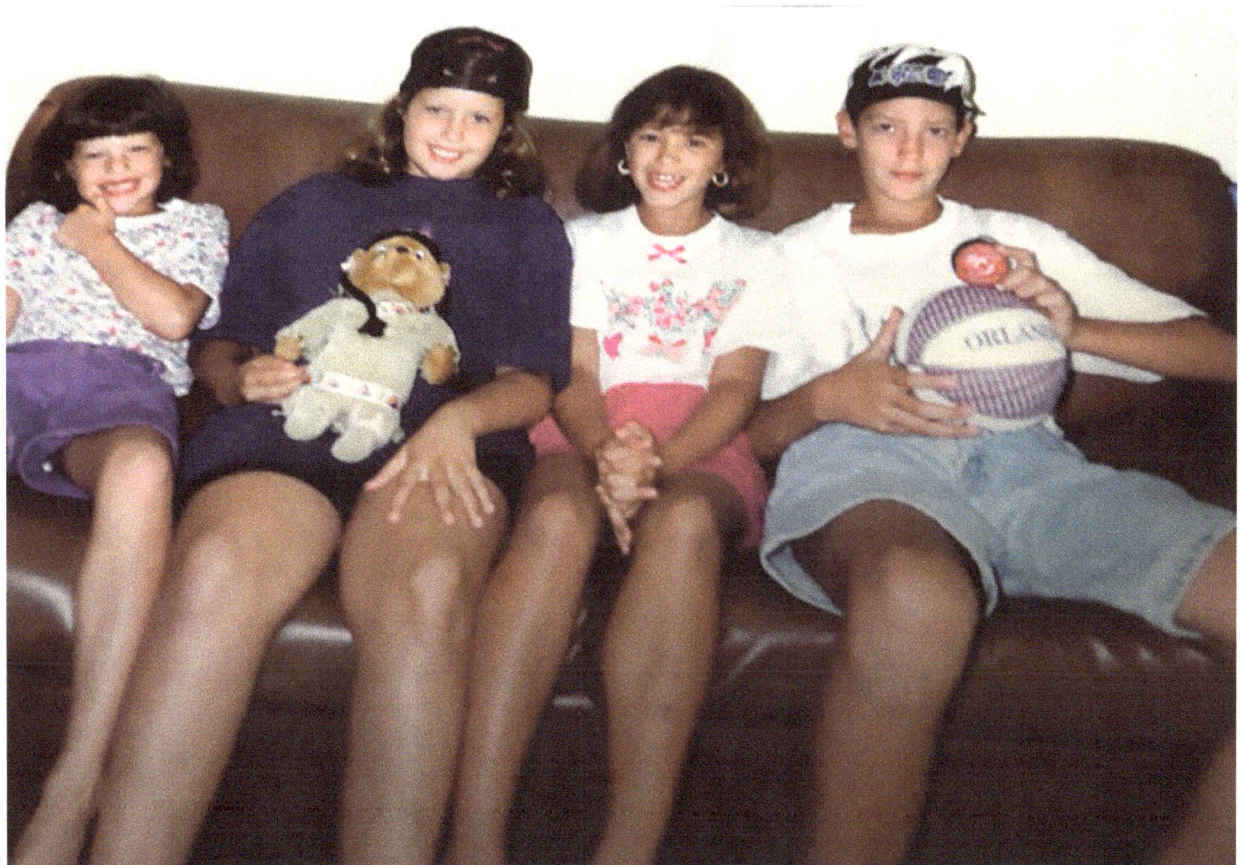

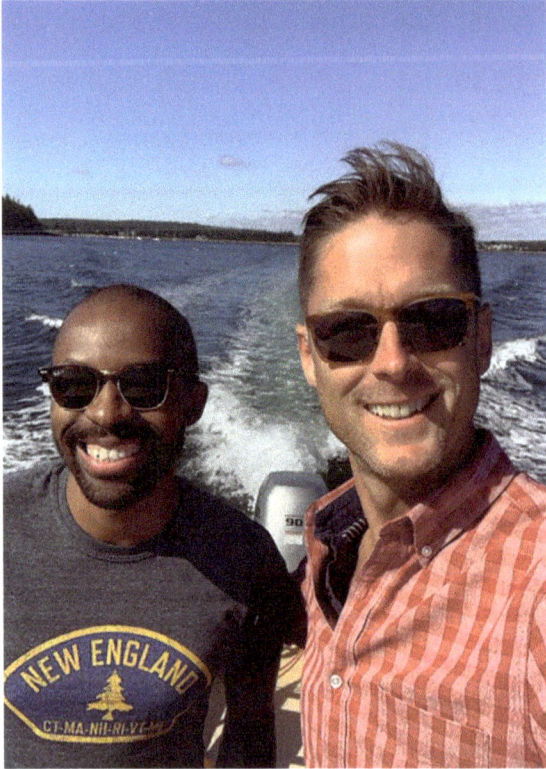

Dallas Dixon
Dementia author and wanna be dementia advocate and activist.
1d · 🌐

Two quick dementia observations 1 It's ok tto move slowly even a lot . Don't let the regulars tell you differently. They can consciously or un consciously bully . 2 My dreams seem more real than everyday life. I seem reluctant to let go of them come morning

😊 ⭕ 2 · 1 comment

👍 Like   💬 Comment   ↗ Share   ✈ Send

Add a comment...   ☺ 🖼

Belinda Mason • 1st   10h •••
Assistant in Nursing

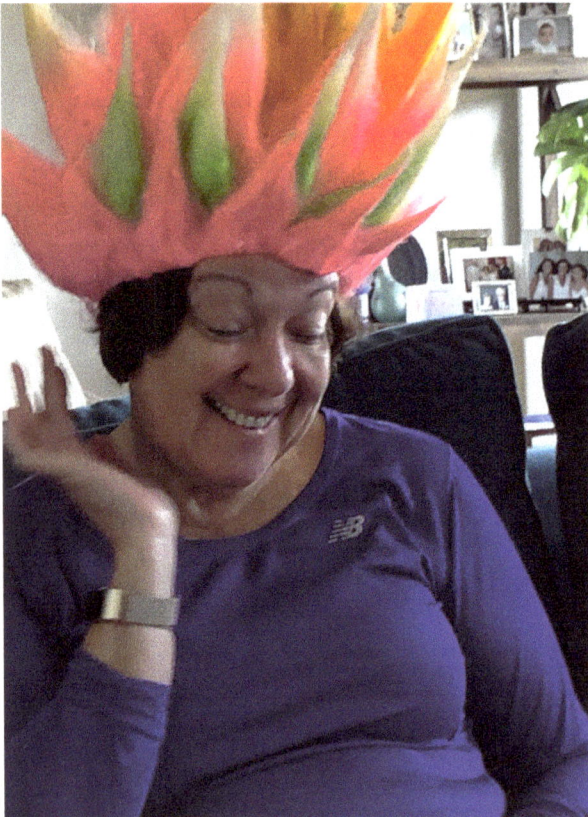

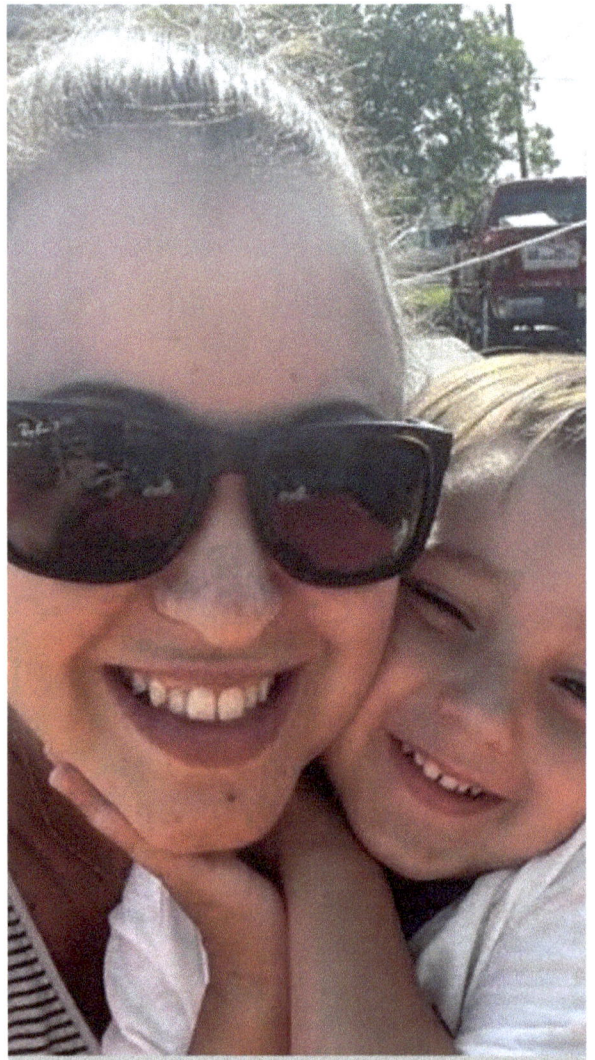

Gina Marie 💕 • 1st
Administrative Assistant
12h

Amen! Thank You Father for ALL You've done and
Continue to Do! ❤️ 🙏

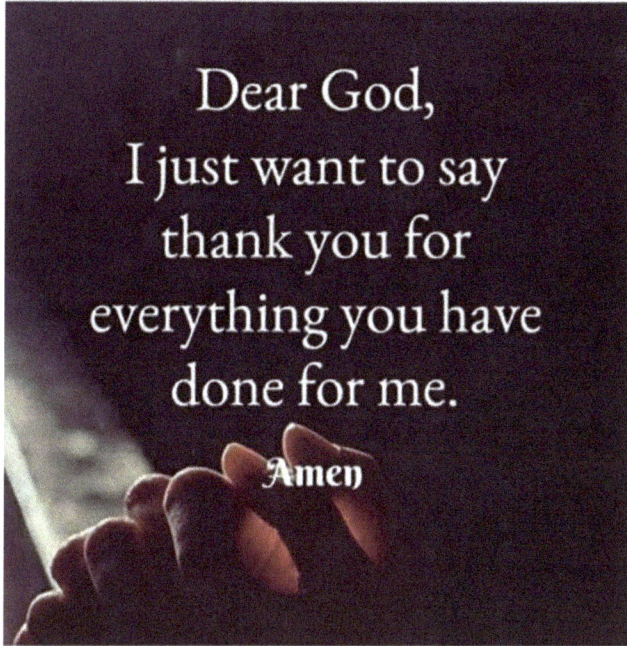

> Dear God,
> I just want to say
> thank you for
> everything you have
> done for me.
> **Amen**

💙❤️💚 92   24 Comments

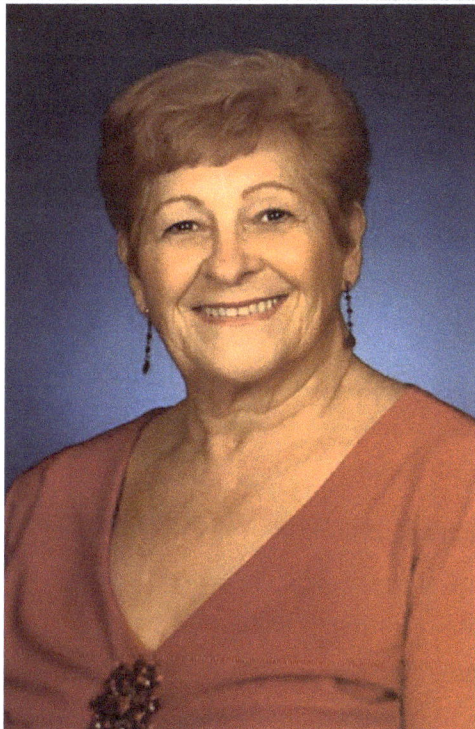

"Those who are certain of the outcome can afford to wait, and wait without anxiety... Patience is natural to those who trust."

A Course in Miracles

Dementia World: There is no shame or pity in forgetting whatever its manifestation.

And remember we don't lose the ability to read your tone and affect.

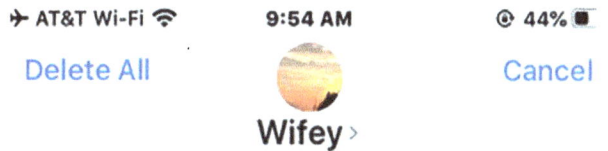

✈ AT&T Wi-Fi 📶   9:54 AM   @ 44% 🔋

Delete All   Cancel

Wifey ›

er to put inthe
basement.... 😍

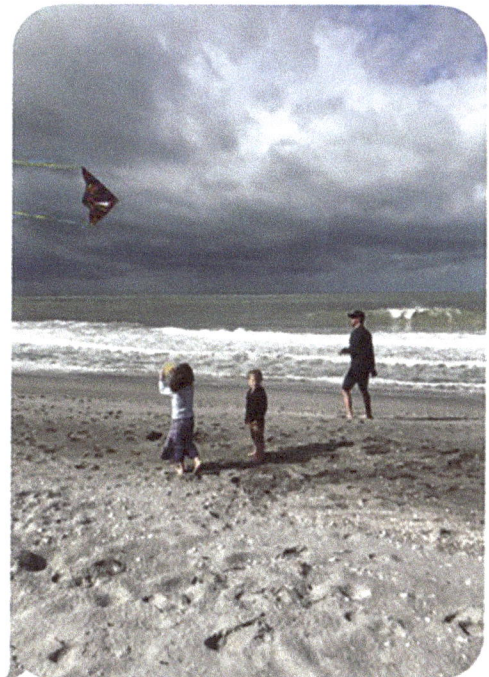

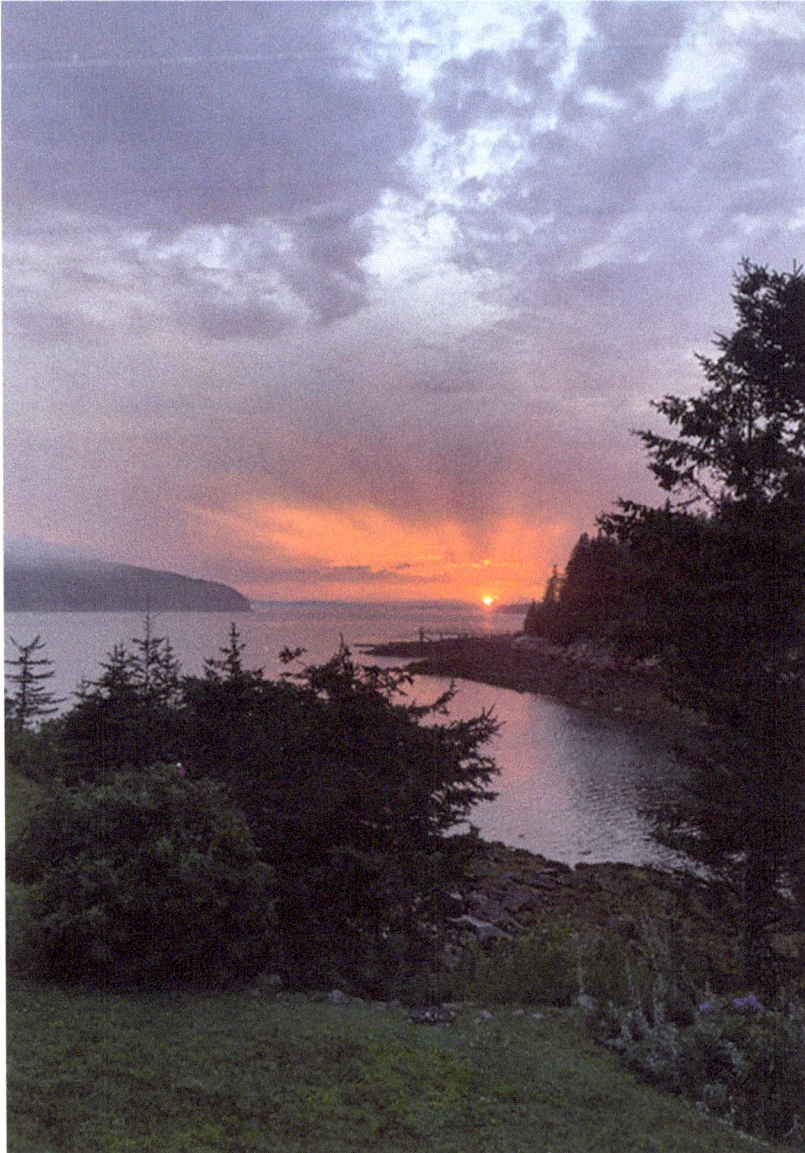

Boycott the Alzheimer's Association until Harry Johns (CEO) issues a warning about the newly publicized Alzheimer's "miracle drug."

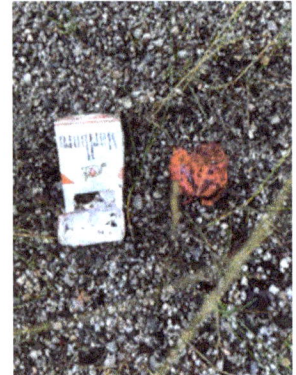

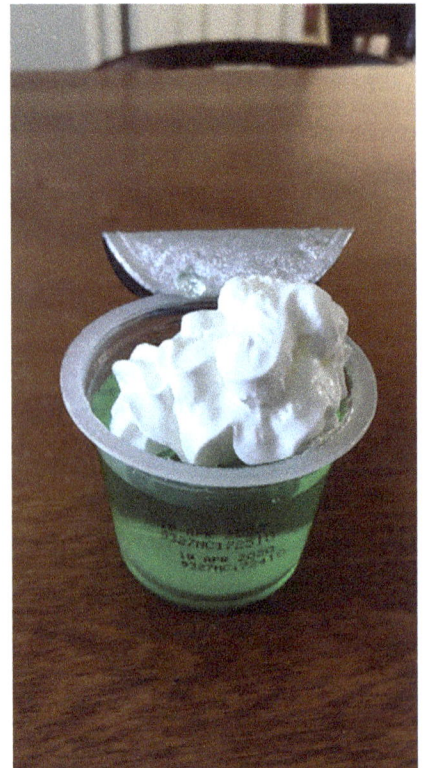

I have been studying about the soul and the spirit. Couldn't understand how they work together. So this came from my God, maybe. The soul is the grandfather clock with all its mechanical pieces. The spirit is time with good-time and bad-time spirits. The creator enabled it all.

May the God of hope
fill you with all joy
and peace as you trust in him,
so that you may overflo
with hope by the power of the
Holy Spirit.

Romans 15:13

Dementia Muse: People equate good friendship with understanding dementia well. Maybe it's just the opposite.

Dementia World: Wake up; a cure is on the horizon.

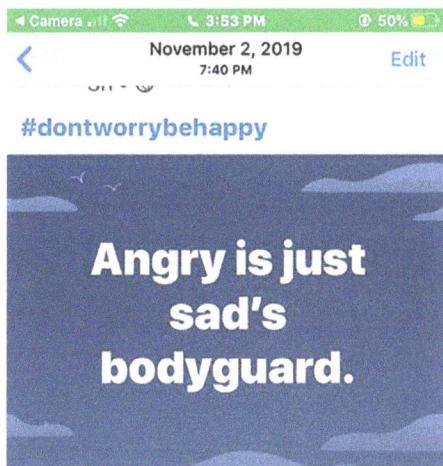

#dontworrybehappy

Angry is just sad's bodyguard.

❤ 3

👍 Like   💬 Comment

↪ Share

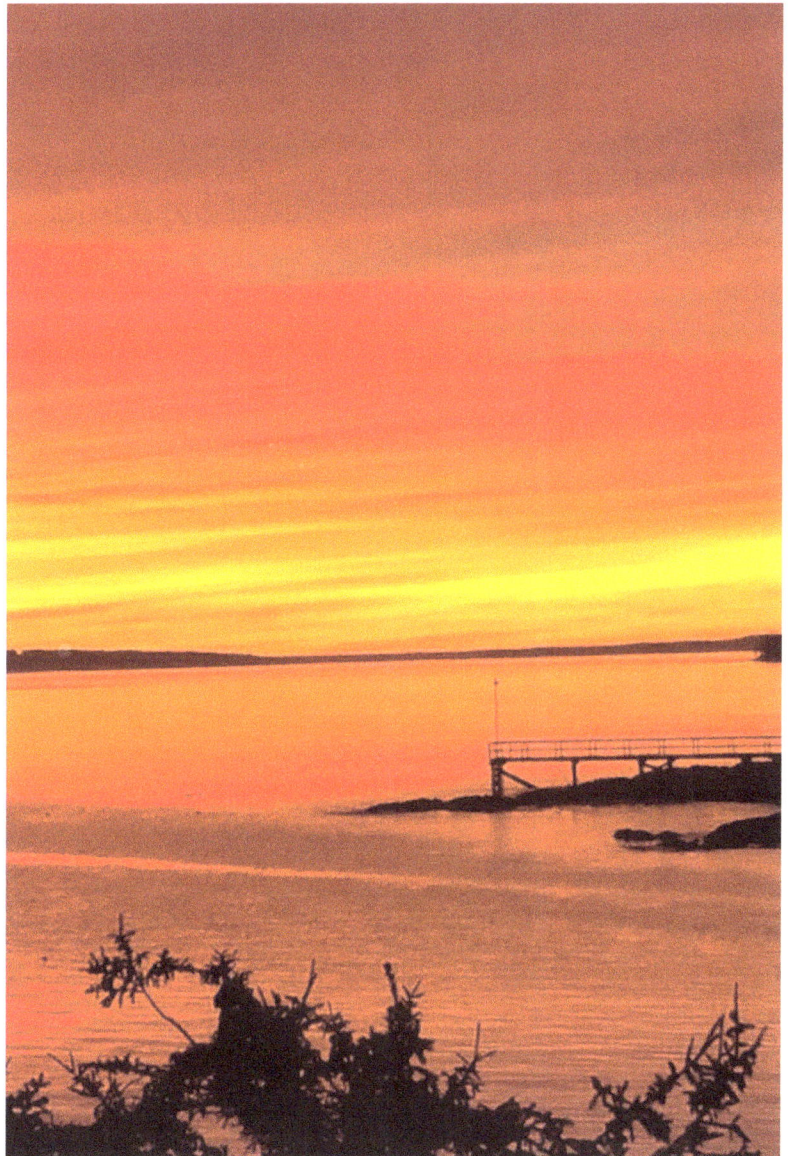

The grace of the Lord Jesus Christ be with your spirit.

Philemon 1:25

In this dude's dementia, music takes the top spot by a mile.

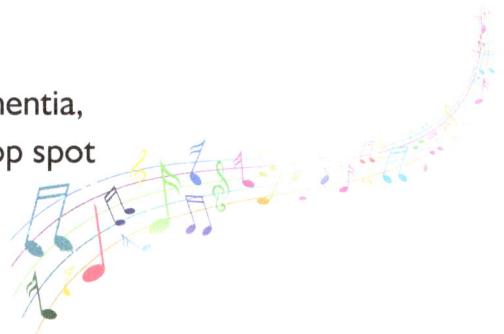

Mount Sinai Won't Administer Aduhelm to Patients

The rejection of the new Alzheimer's drug by the two major medical centers is one of the starkest signs of concern over its approval by the F.D.A.

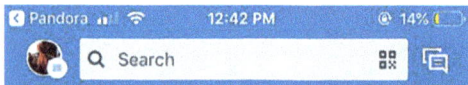

🔍 Search   ⊞⊟ 🗨

✏️ Write a post   📹 📷

🟡 **Hannah Tucker** • 1st
   RCFE-Gerontology Student looking for work
   1h   • • •

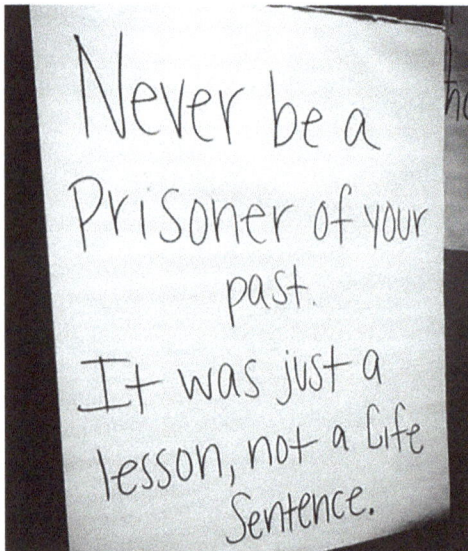

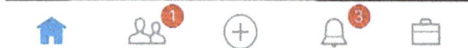

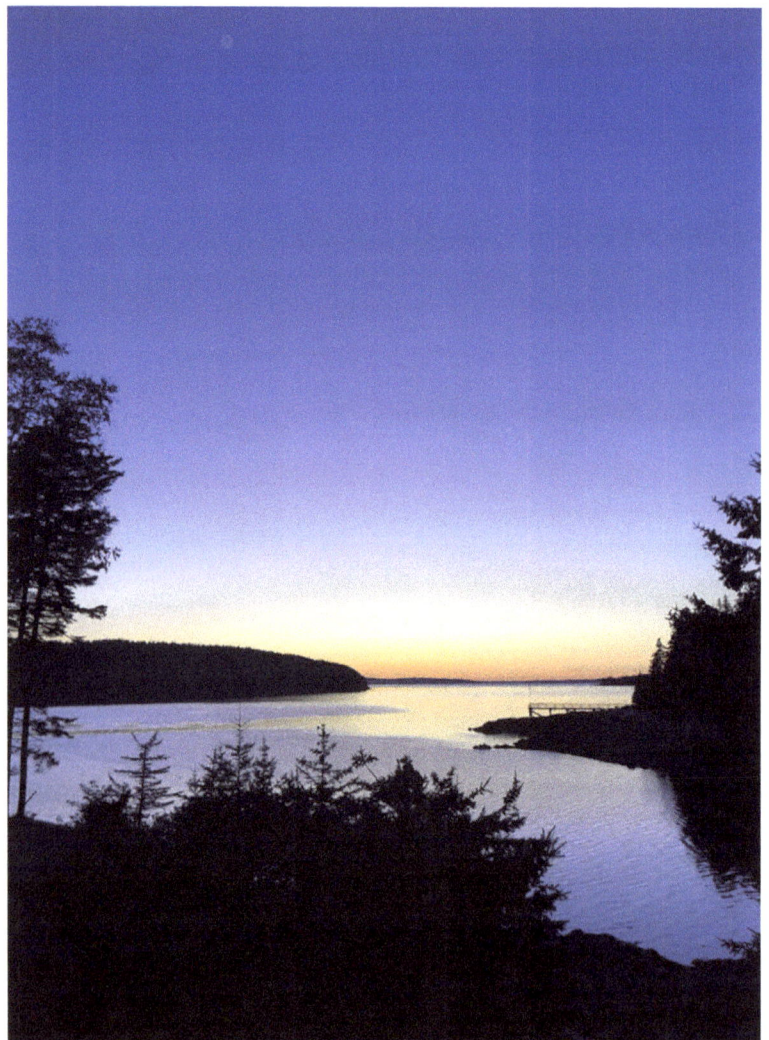

Never be a Prisoner of your past. It was just a lesson, not a life Sentence.

🏠   👥①   ⊕   🔔③   💼

If my memory is correct (lol) the Alzheimer's Association raved about this new drug. Shame on you for your premature ejaculation. The only organization that acted with responsible response was DAI (Dementia Alliance International), which is for us and run by us dementia dudettes and dudes. Kate Swaffer

Mount Sinai Won't Administer Aduhelm to Patients
The rejection of the new Alzheimer's drug by the two major medical centers is one of the starkest signs of concern over its approval by the F.D.A.

Lobster Price June 22 Retail, Ellsworth Area
$9.99 per pound (small)
$11.99 per pound (large)

front

Baked then boiled

Study examines effect of THC on lobsters

By ETHAN GENTER
SOUTHWEST HARBOR — Charlotte's Legendary Lobster Pound lived up to its name when owner Charlotte Gill made international headlines for her attempts to find a more humane way to cook lobsters by exposing them to marijuana smoke. Now, a few years later, here's some science behind it.

In 2018, Gill, with the help of an air mattress pump, funneled smoke from her homegrown marijuana into a sealed container that held a lobster in equal parts water and air. would then hotbox the for three to five minfully sedating them so the cooking process would etically be less painful. like non-hotboxed lobwhen they went into the Gill said her lobsters barely move, indicating

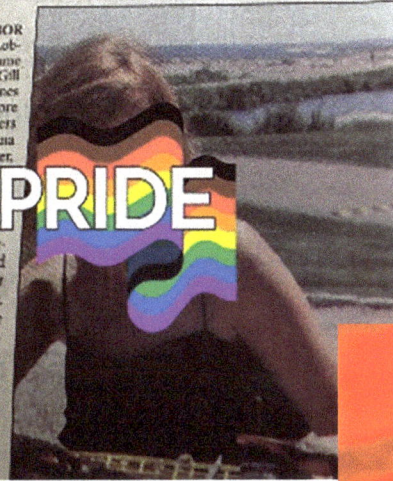

PRIDE

STUDY EXAMINES EFFECT OF THC ON LOBSTERS
It must be hard rolling a joint
with those claws.

U know what's sorta interesting within our dementia world? The longer the time dementia has blessed my life, the less important is the mess the medical world calls diagnosis or "cure." For me, it ultimately comes down to if I had a choice to go back, I wouldn't go back.

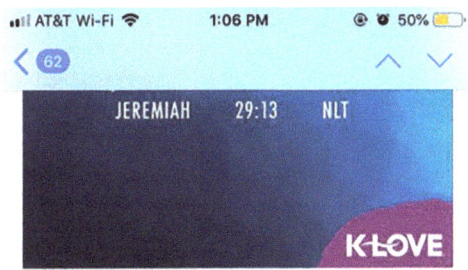

.ıll AT&T Wi-Fi 📶 1:06 PM @ ☉ 50% 🔋

< 62 ∧ ∨

JEREMIAH 29:13 NLT

K-LOVE

8/30/2019

If you look for me wholeheartedly, you will find me.

Jeremiah 29:13 (NLT) View in Context

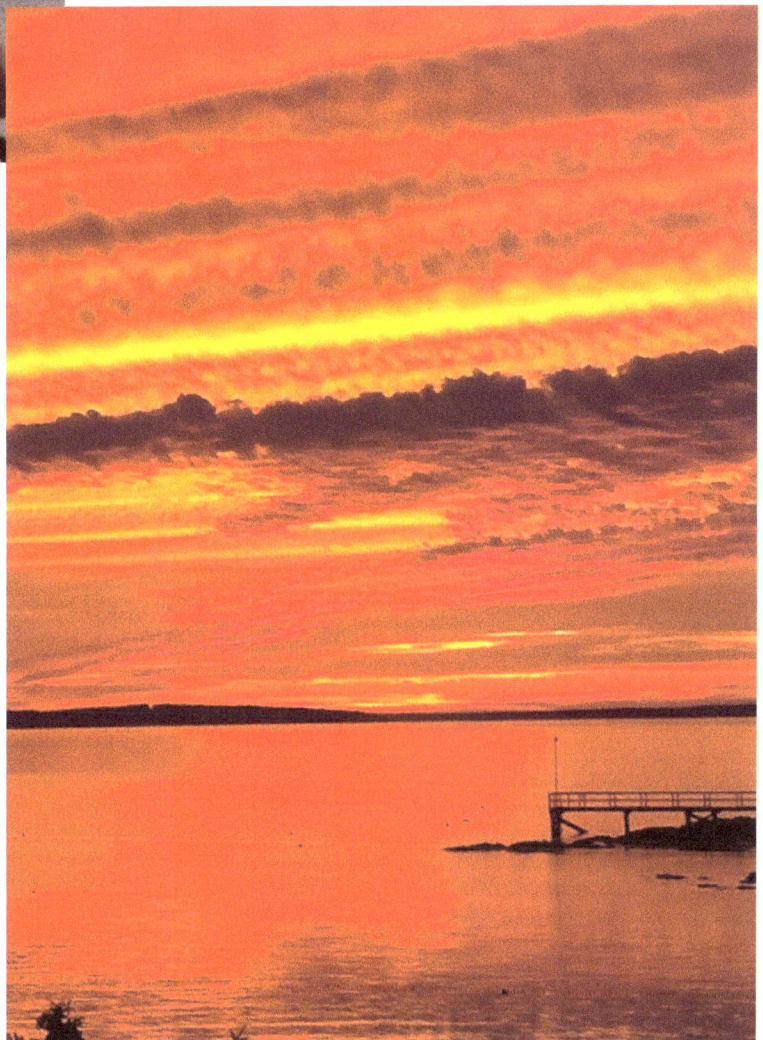

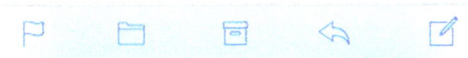

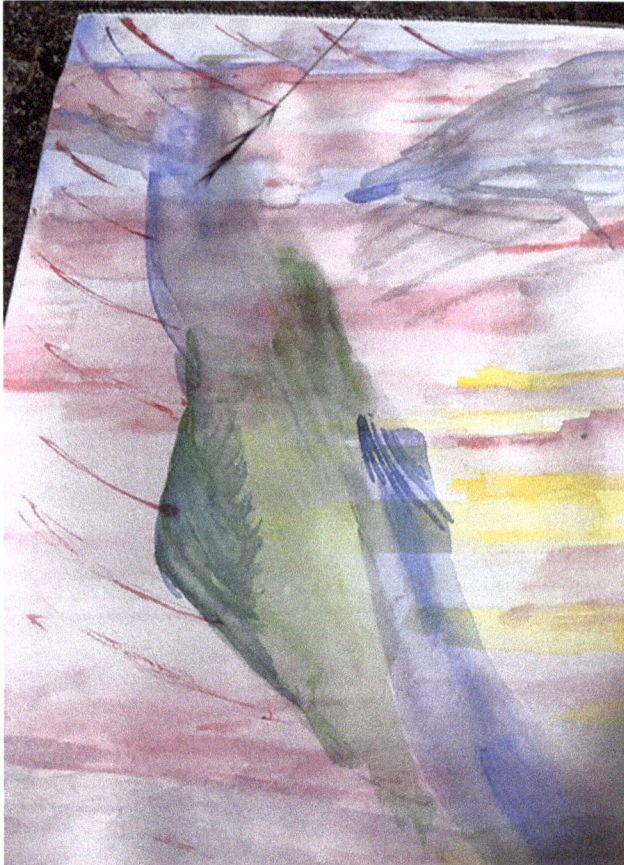

QUICK DEMENTIA OBSERVATION:

When we say something tongue in cheek, it may be received as

DEMENTIAFRIED.

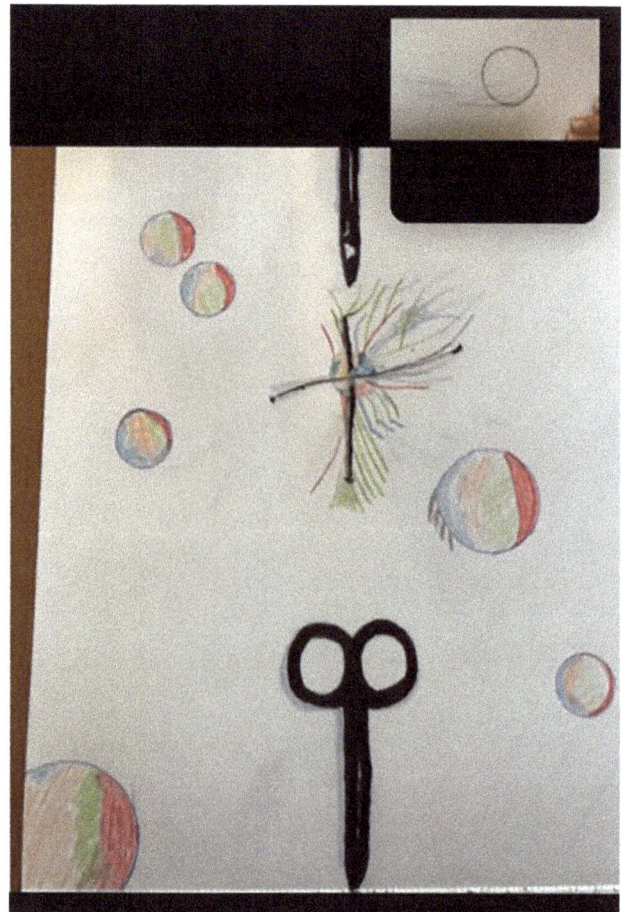

August 2020

It must drive regular people nuts when us demented flit from one thing to another, without enough time on task. Don't believe it.

Flitting is so cool.

Regs would be jealous if they knew.

See what great love the Father has lavished on us, that we should be called children of God! And that is what we are! The reason the world does not know us is that it did not know him.

1 John 3:1

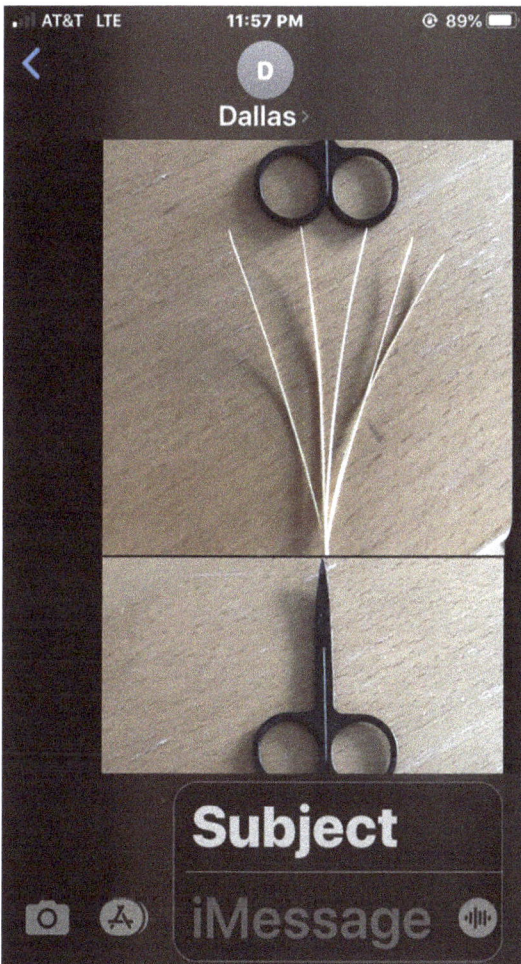

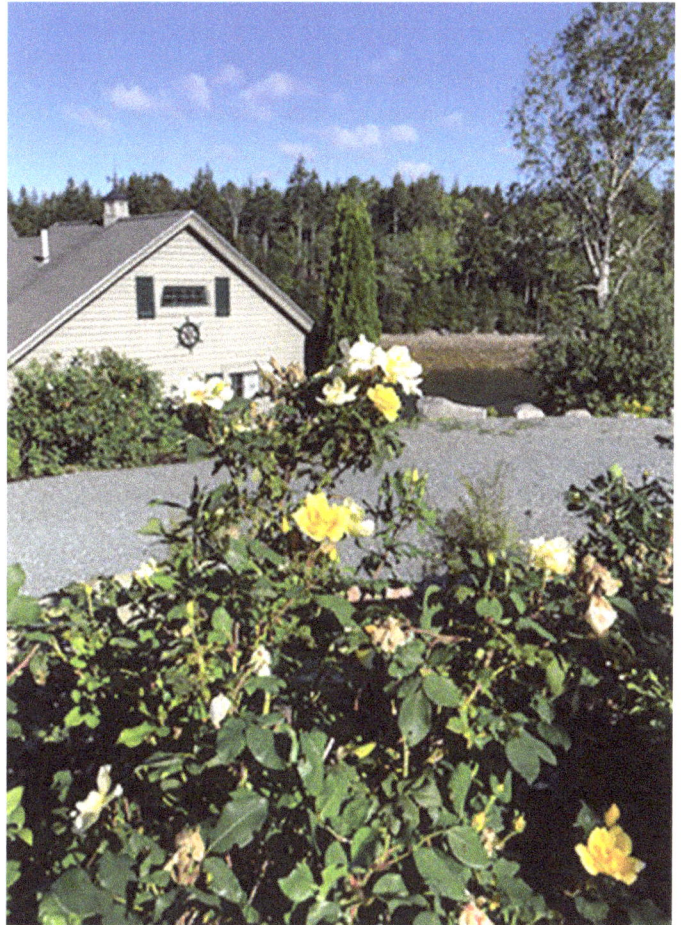

"So you say dementia is a blessing, dementia dude? And tell me about this blessing." If God looks to refine us all as better souls through both trial and blessing, why would dementia be different? And a God blessing, even one from God, is so, so amazingly divine that we need not count them . . . or even remember them but for a moment . . . to give thanks. Dear Lord, I am thankful for my dementia. Strengthen those around me whose life has been burdened.
Bless them.

January 2021

The various "stages of dementia" theory folks have taught us with their normal people biases. Made all of dementia people dead on arrival. Stages mean death is close at hand, even though that is not true for us. Our "progression" is a seemingly wonderful way to die, even with all of death's tangles notwithstanding.

Maybe it's just a getting old.

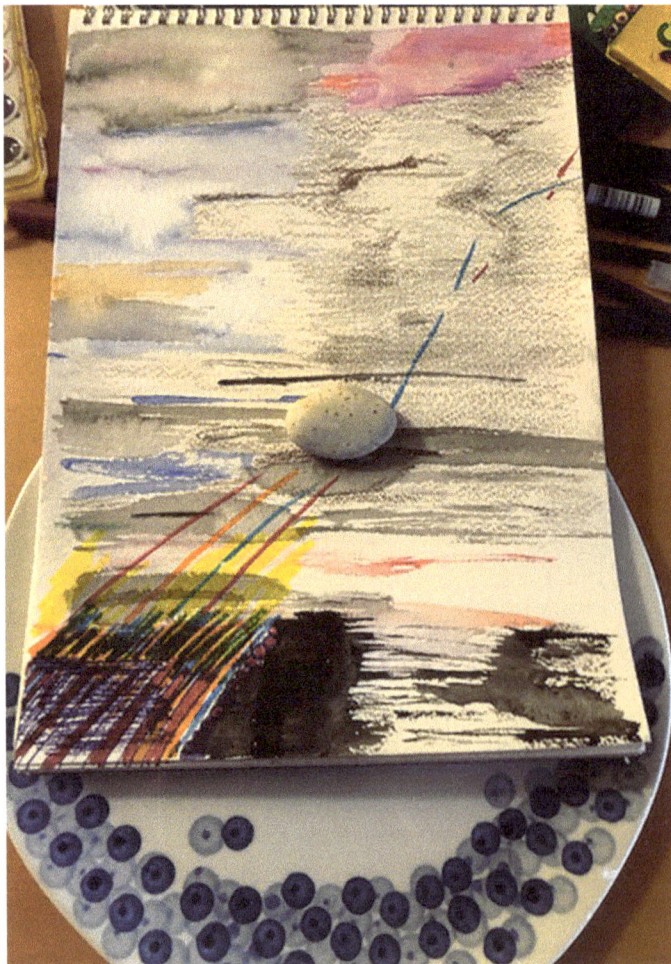

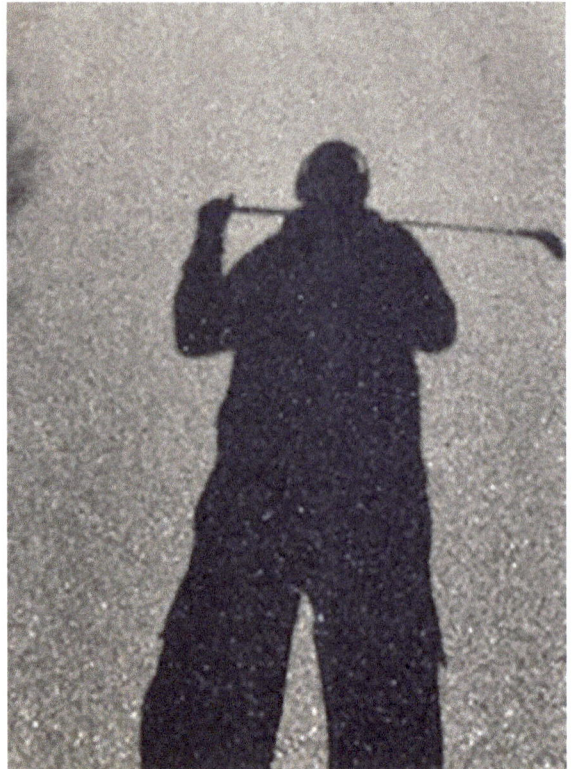

"Dallas Dixon is the irreverent Dementia Dude. He posts insightful and witty commentary on his LinkedIn profile about dementia. Dallas said that at first, he looked for diagnostic answers and found Teepa Snow. She was, "the only normal person who knew dementia and truly liked us. Heavenly!"

Kathleen Landel, MA,
PAC Mentor

I know this truth firsthand: guilt frenzies the soul; grace calms it. The benefit of being a great sinner is dependence upon a great grace!

Thank you, God!

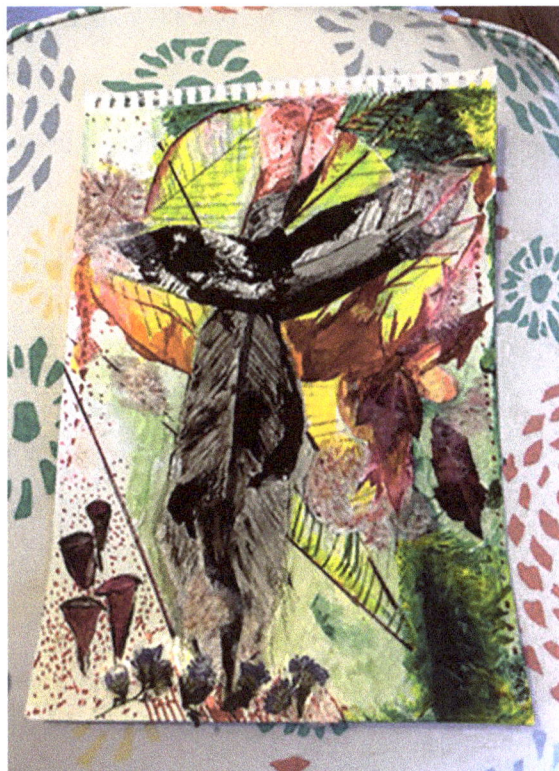

of 5 Thayer brothers, Cape May, NJ 1898

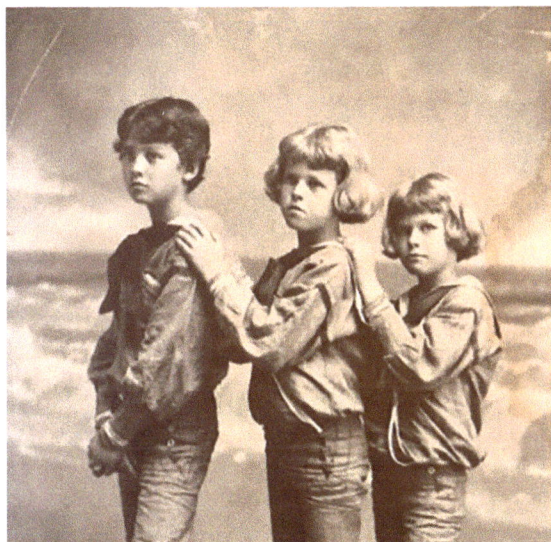

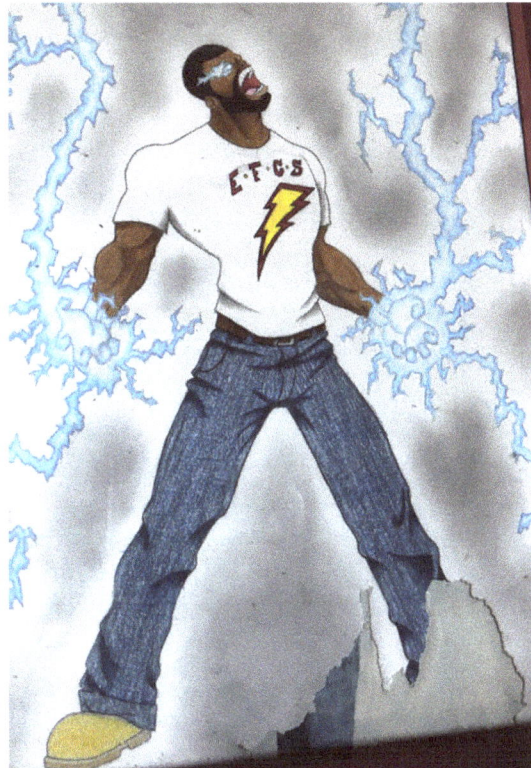

by Emil Fennel

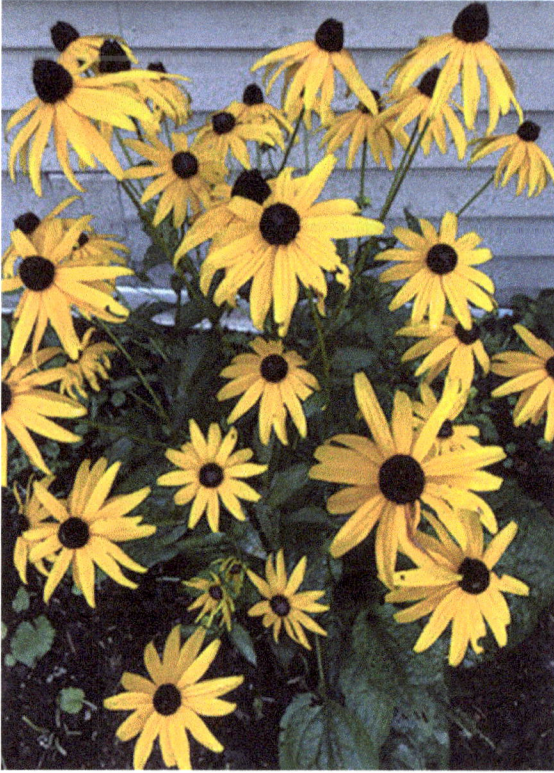

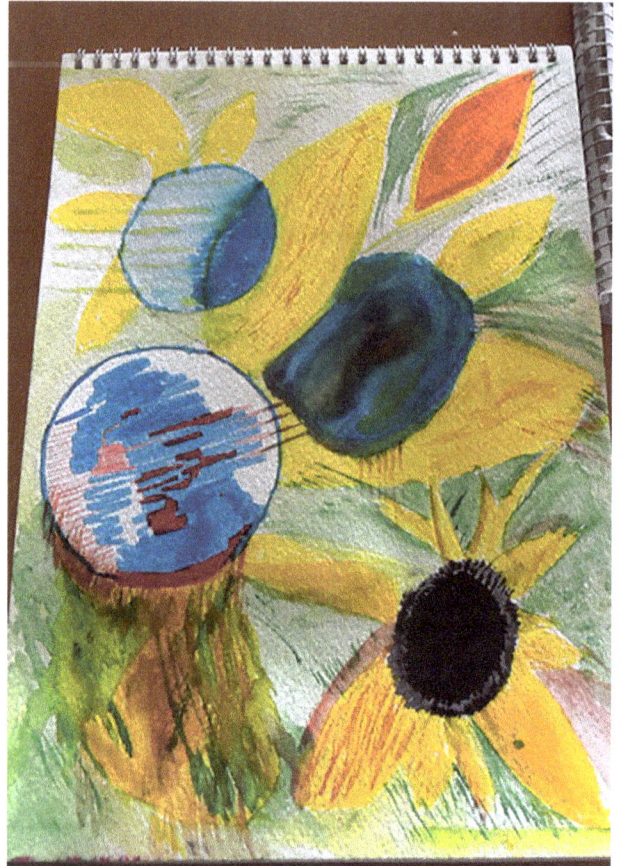

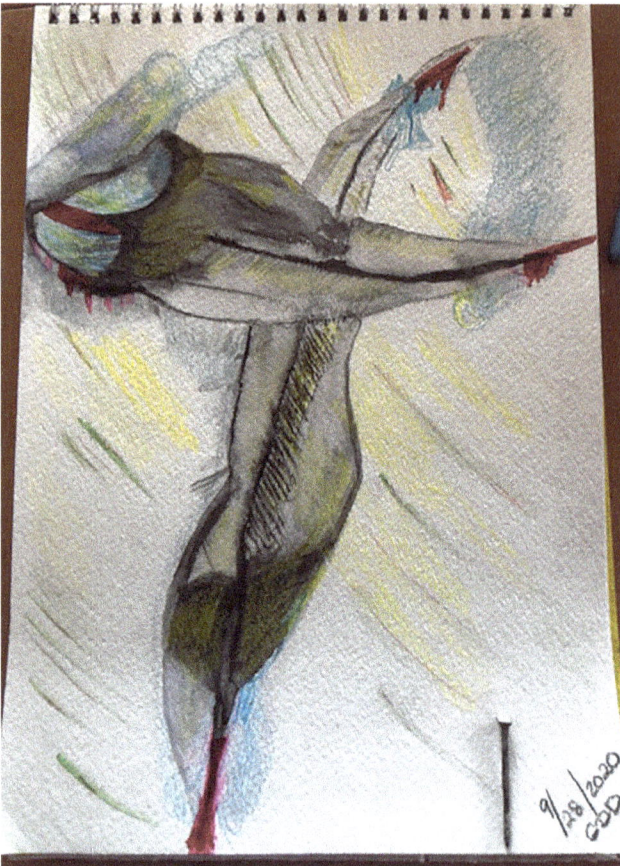

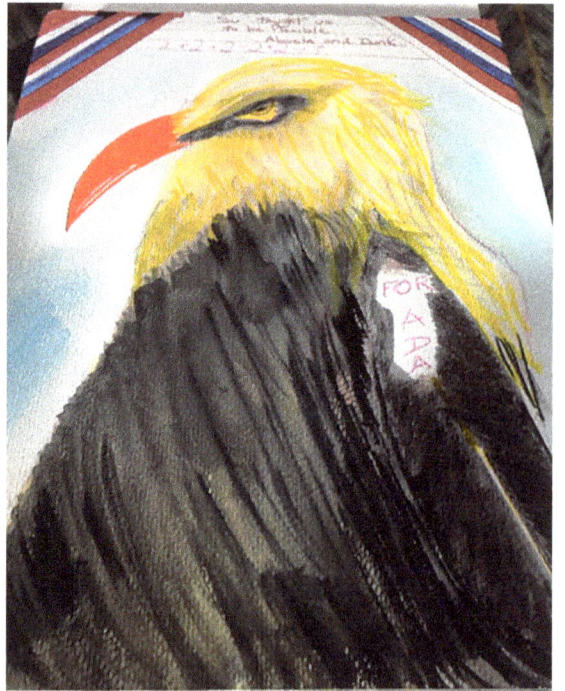

46

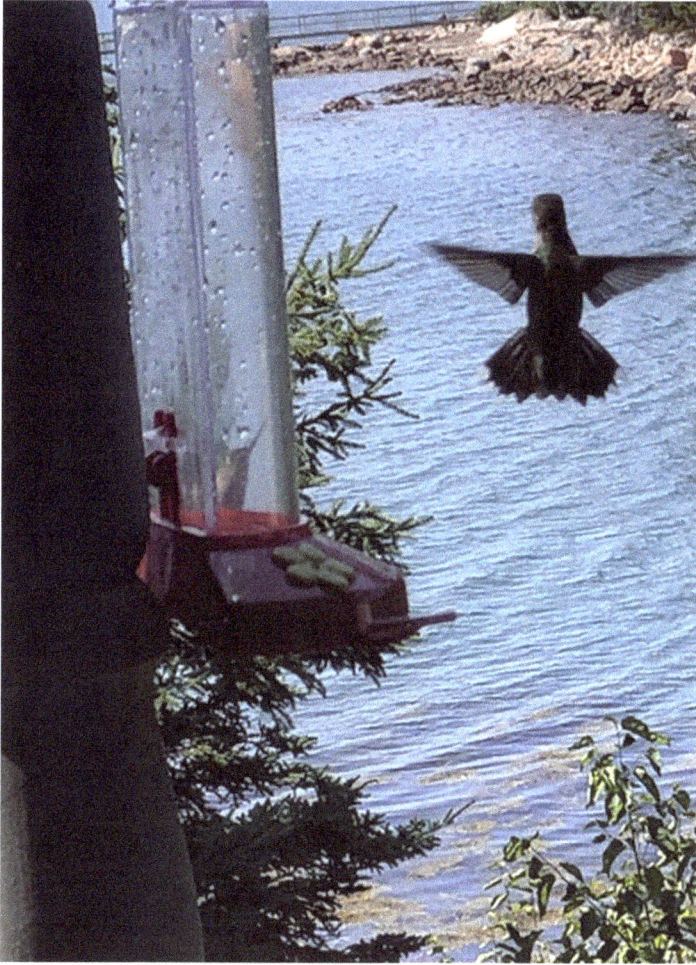

August 2021:

As a dementia dude,
I can feel my world,
my brain slowing down.

I like it.

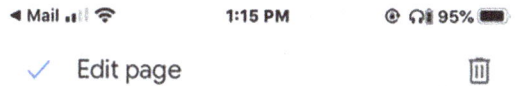
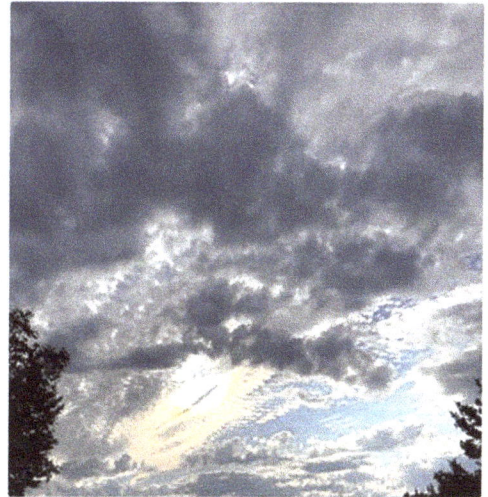

January 2021

Another amazing little symptom . . . popped up. A regular asks you a question and you (trying to be a regular person) want to answer at a regular person's pace. Unable to keep up, you just say something off topic to ease the tension, only to find out you sound a little psycho.

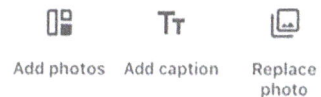

Blogger Gail Gregory asks, "Am I Too Young for Dementia?" Read more about this week's featured author on AlzAuthors.com.
https://lnkd.in
...see more

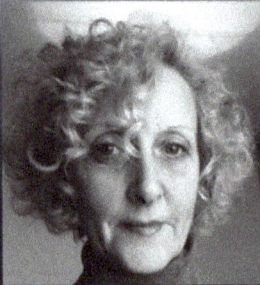

Gail Gregory, blogger at Too Young for Dementia?

I suppose at first when I started writing
I used my writing as a release. This was
a way to get my frustrations out
I then realised I was documenting
something quite special,
this was a new chapter in my life.
This was a New beginning
This was My Dementia Chapter.

AlzAuthors.com

👍 4

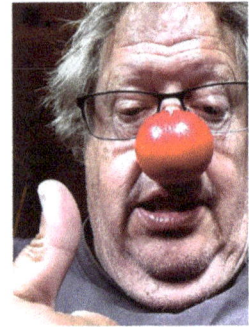

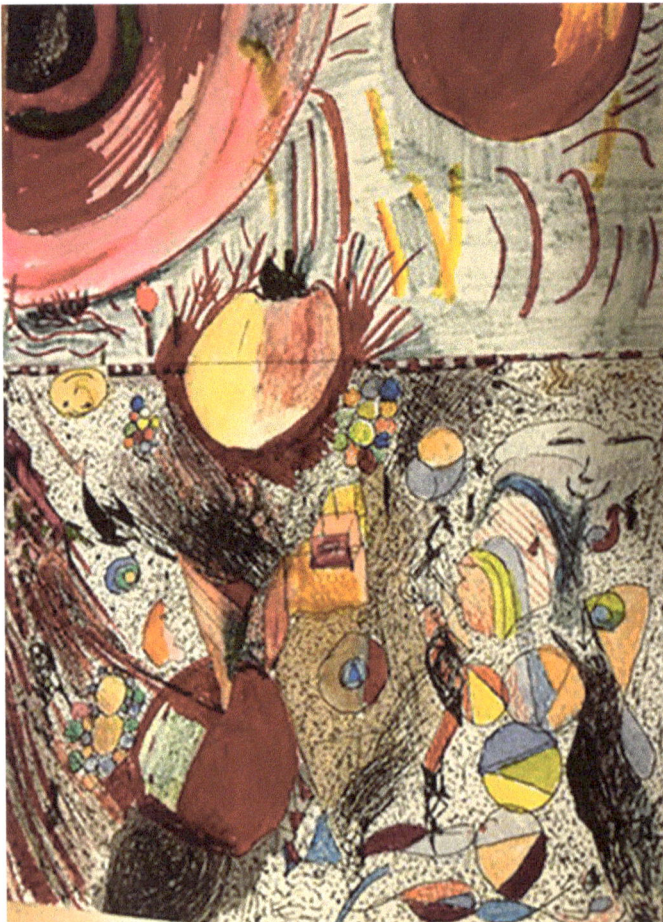

.ıll AT&T 🤏   6:26 PM   🎧 54% 🔋

📷   *Instagram*   ✈

dallasdixon7

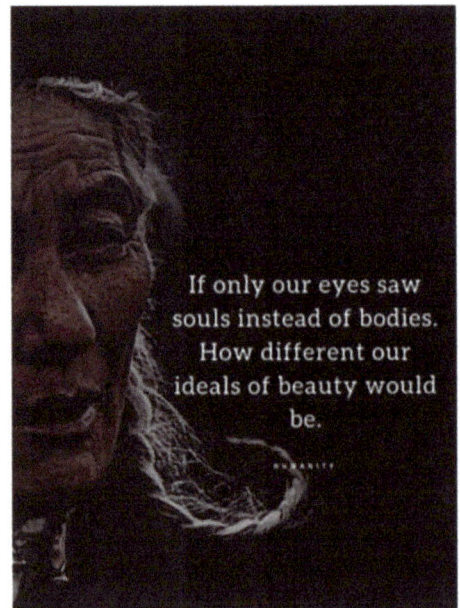

If only our eyes saw
souls instead of bodies.
How different our
ideals of beauty would
be.

HUMANITY

👍 13

♡ Q ✈   🔖

3 likes

🏠   🔍   ⊕   ♡   👤

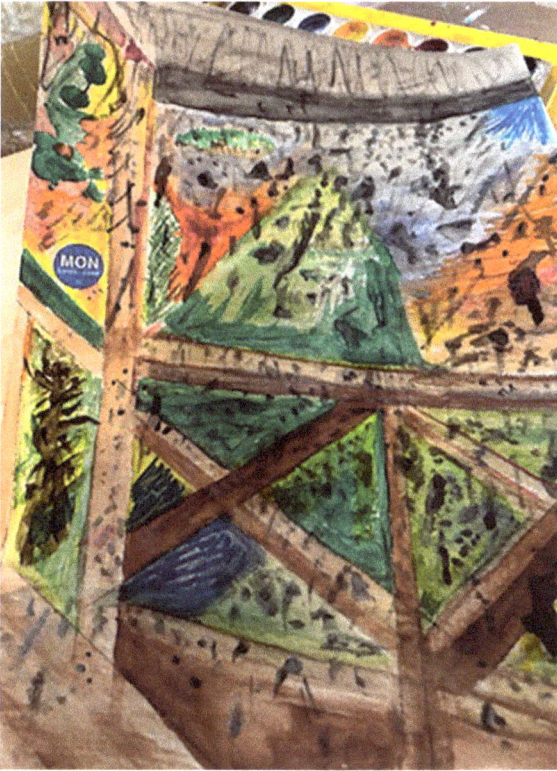
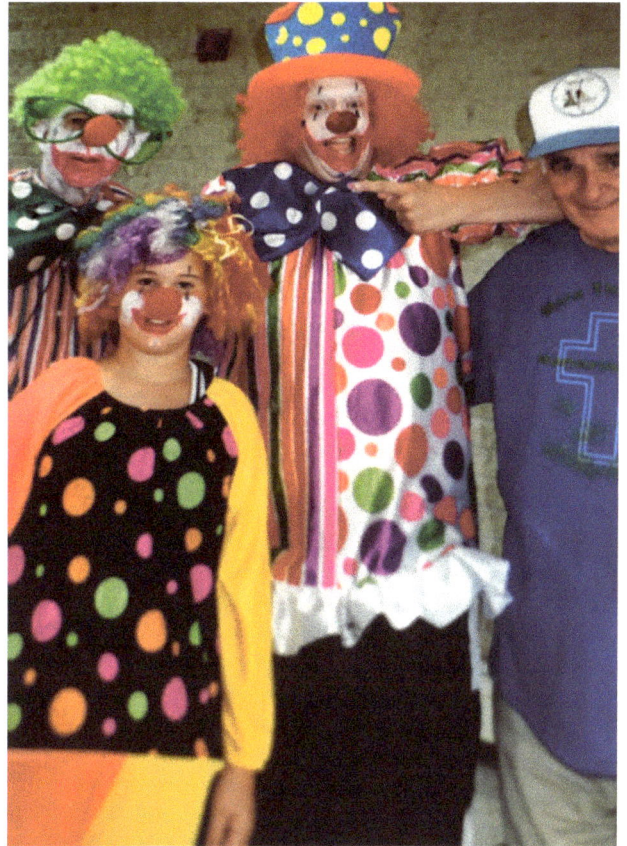
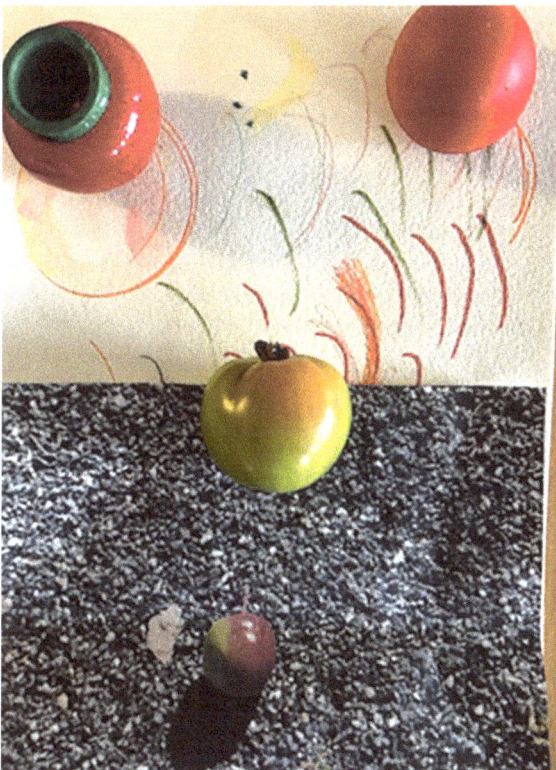
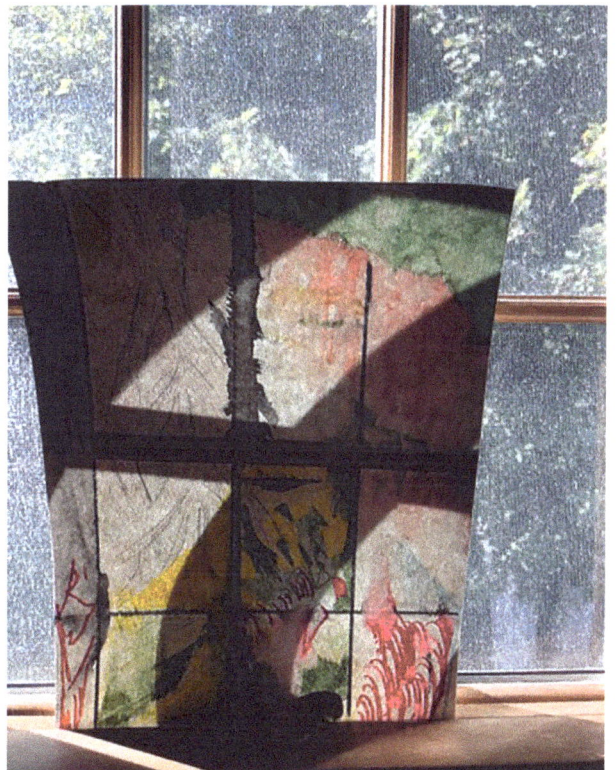

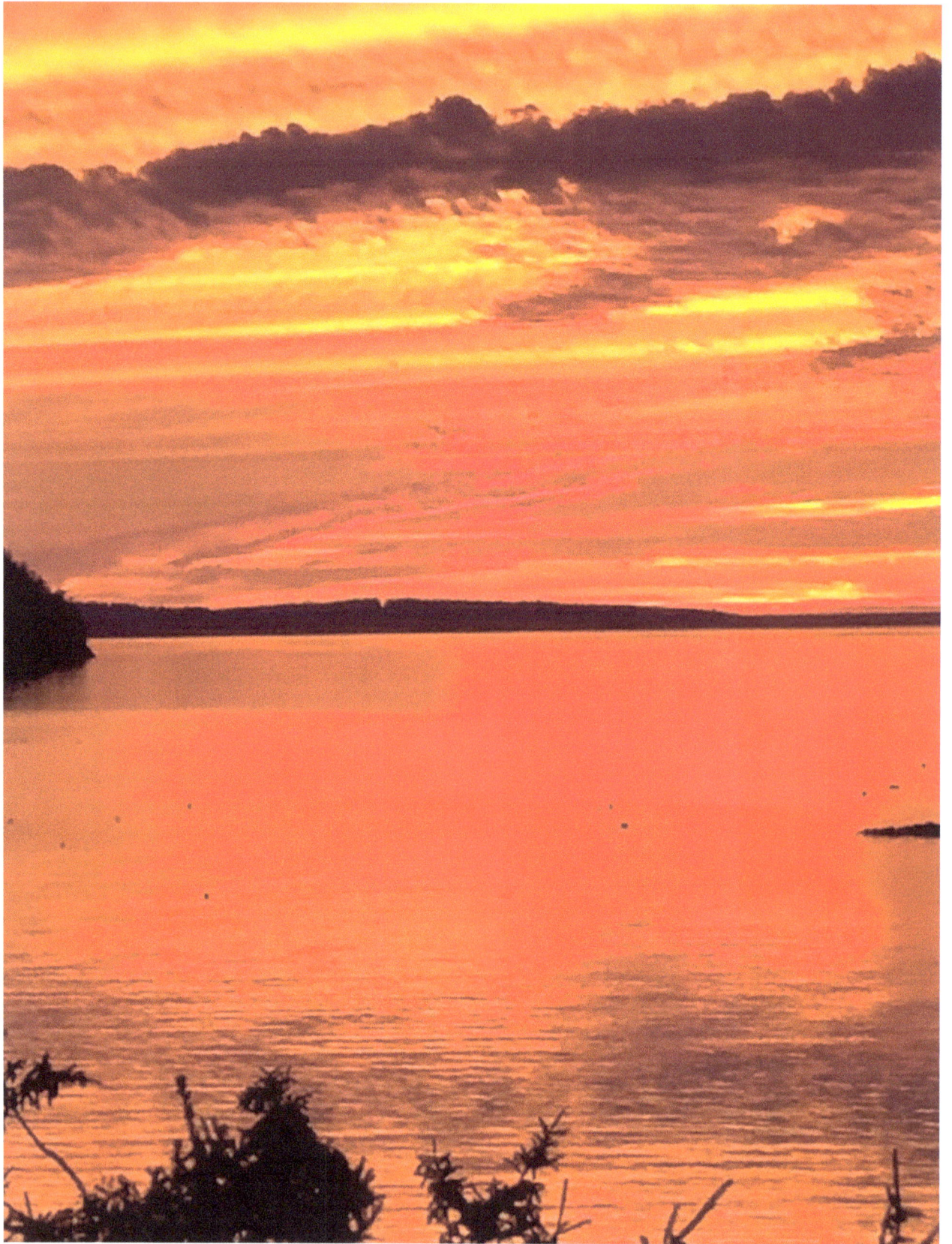

solve crime.

The fatal stabbing happened around 9:50 p.m. Saturday. Patrol officers arrived shortly thereafter and found 33-year-old Daniel Alvaranga, in the intersection of Brunswick Avenue and Southard Street.

He was stabbed in the chest and taken to the hospital, where he was pronounced dead a short time later, the Mercer County Prosecutor's Office said.

The difference between dementia perspectives: Before dementia
, I was a trial lawyer.I pulled Perry Mason - the old infamous trial lawyer drama as a result of conversation with friends at D A I , the only dementia organization run by and for us .. . I couldn't follow it . Some would say tragic ;I say funny. Oh ps it wasn't the show

February 2021

If you are in the dementia world, you know that the new COVID strain is easier to catch. And if you add in that us dementia folks are at least twice as likely to contract the virus, you might think we are concerned.

Nah. I figure we'll just wear 5-and-1/2 masks.

Should do it.

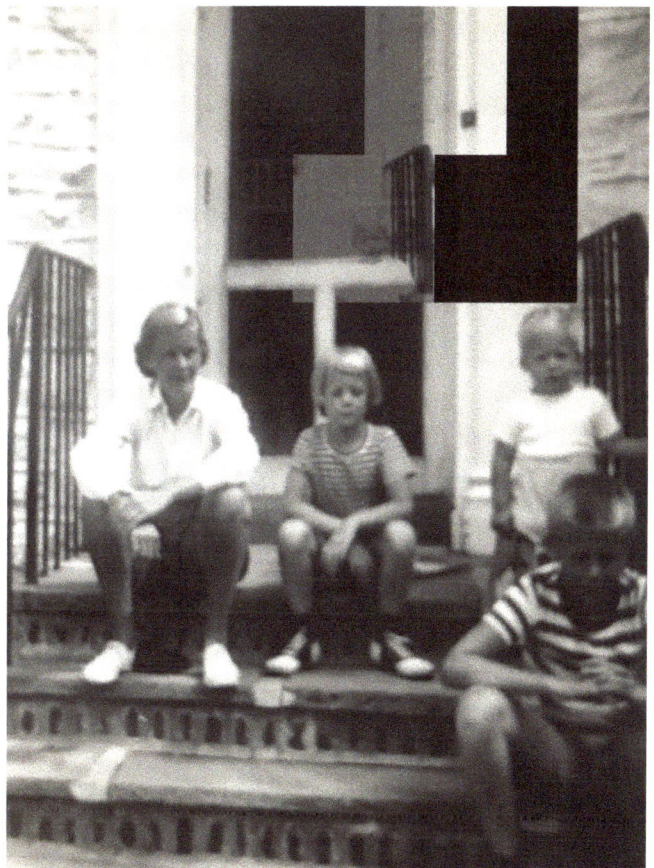

verse of the Day

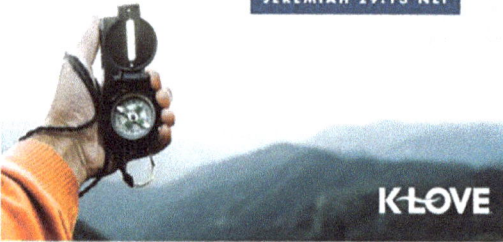

K-LOVE

IF YOU LOOK FOR ME WHOLEHEARTEDLY, YOU WILL FIND ME.

JEREMIAH 29:13 NLT

K-LOVE

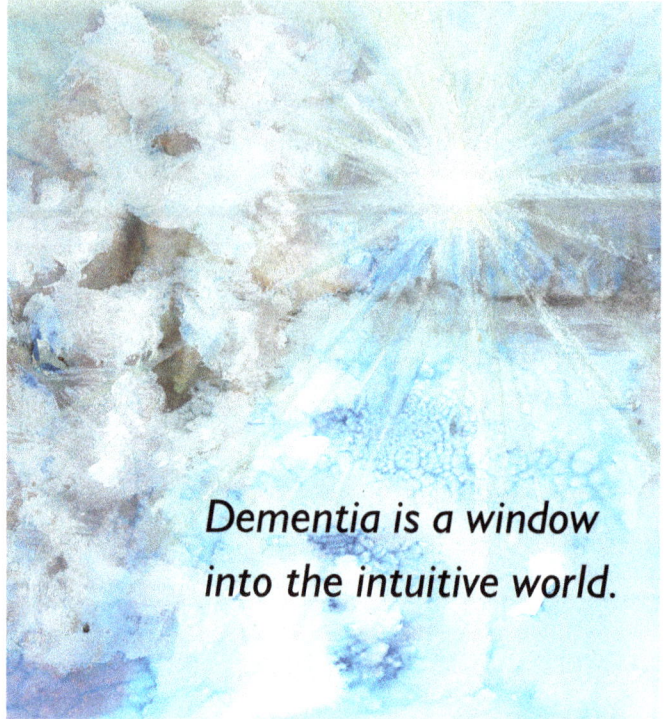

Dementia is a window into the intuitive world.

Let no debt remain outstanding, except the continuing debt to love one another, for whoever loves others has fulfilled the law.

Romans 13:8

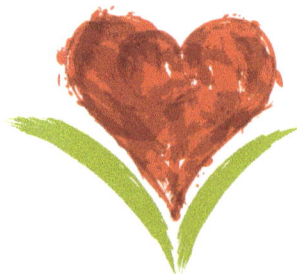

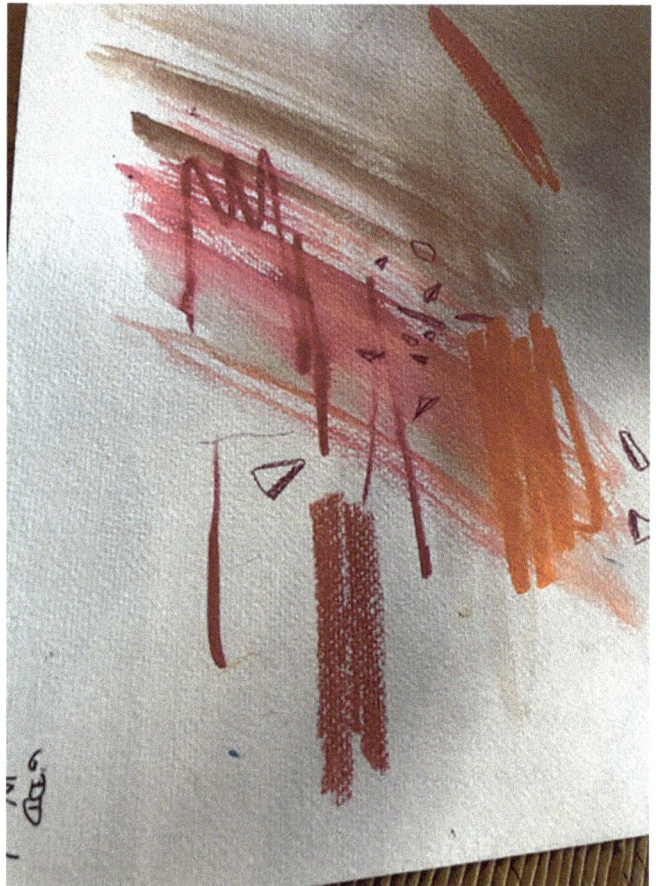

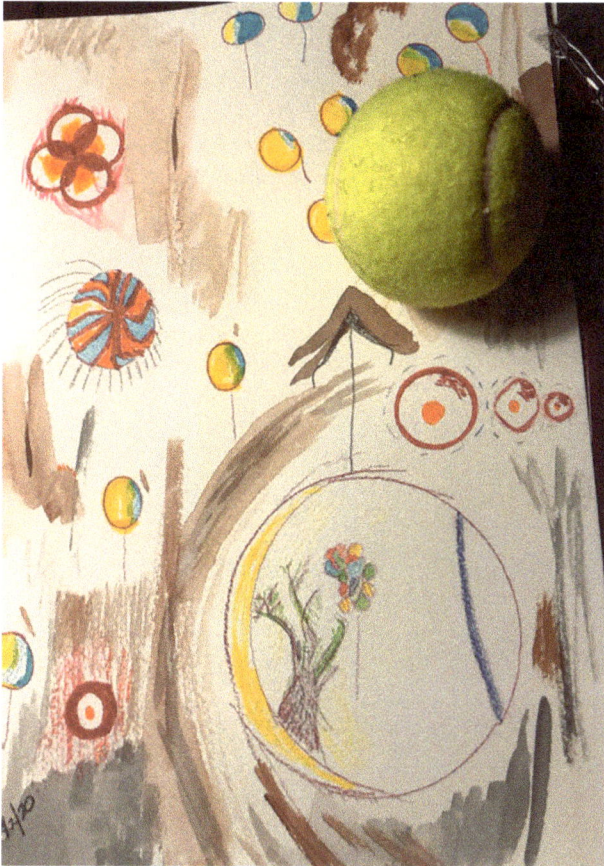

Demetia Dog

The Dementia Dog . . . A Superhero for every Dementia dude and dudette and every organization.

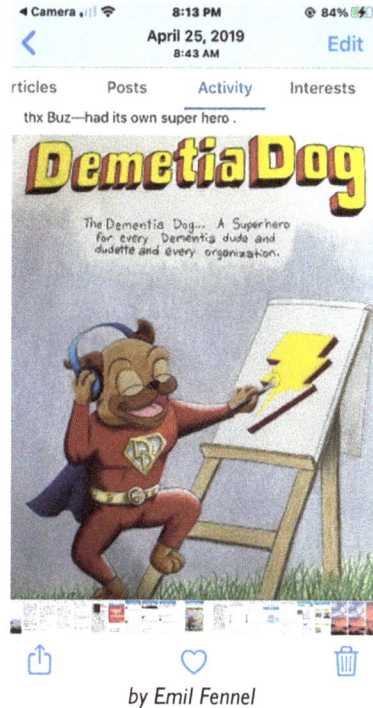

by Emil Fennel

February 2021 – Just sayin'.

People with dementia have significantly greater risk of contracting the coronavirus and are much more likely to be hospitalized and die from it, than people without dementia do, a new study of millions of medical records in the United States has found.

Their risk could not be entirely explained by characteristics common to people with dementia that are known risk factors for Covid-19: old age, living in a nursing home, and having conditions like obesity, asthma, diabetes and cardiovascular disease. After researchers adjusted those factors, Americans with dementia were still twice as likely to have gotten Covid-19 as of late last summer.

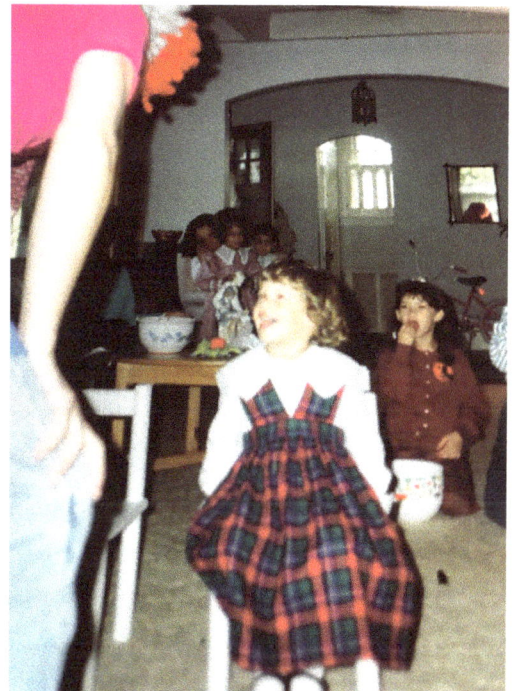

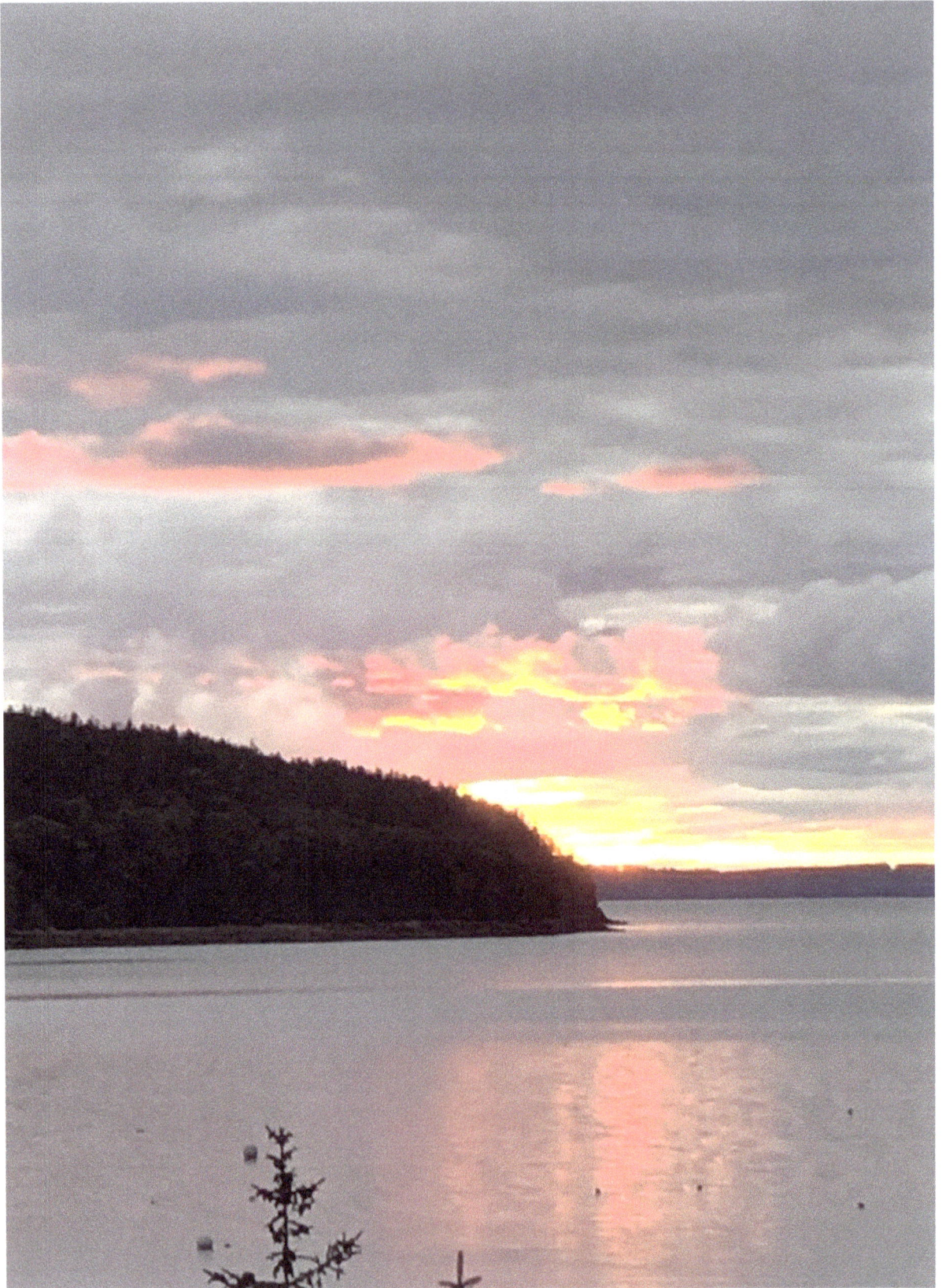

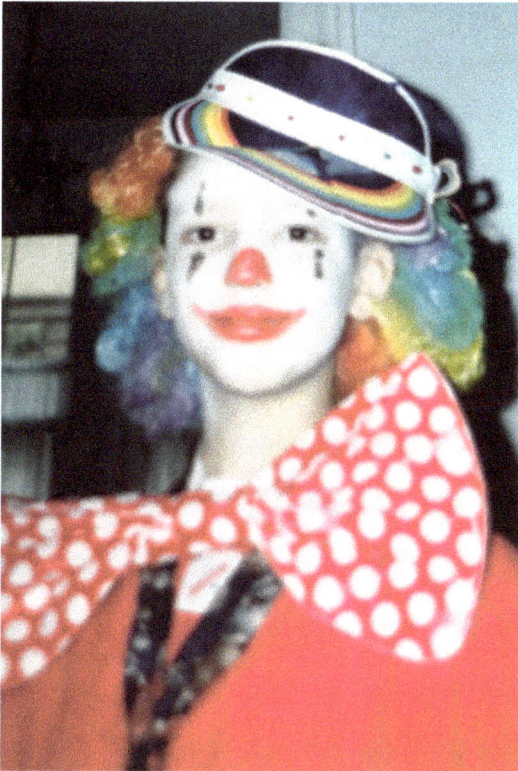

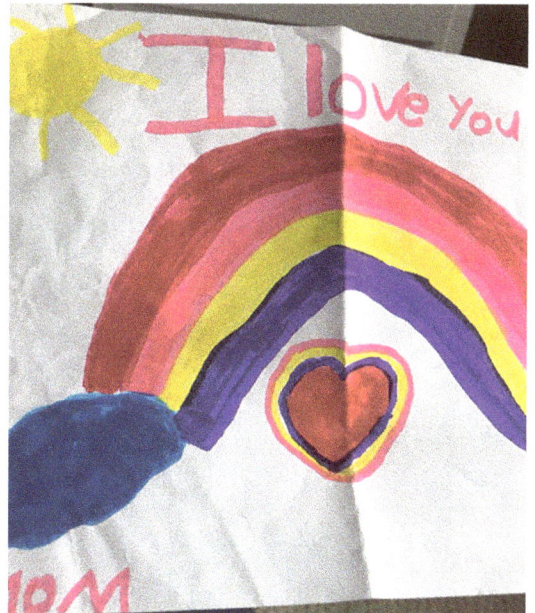

*Love is patient, love is kind.
It does not envy, it does not boast,
it is not proud. It does not dishonor
others, it is not self-seeking, it is not
easily angered, it keeps no record
of wrongs.*
1 Corinthians 13:4-5

*And so we know and rely on the love
God has for us. God is love. Whoever
lives in love lives in God, and God
in them.*
1 John 4:16

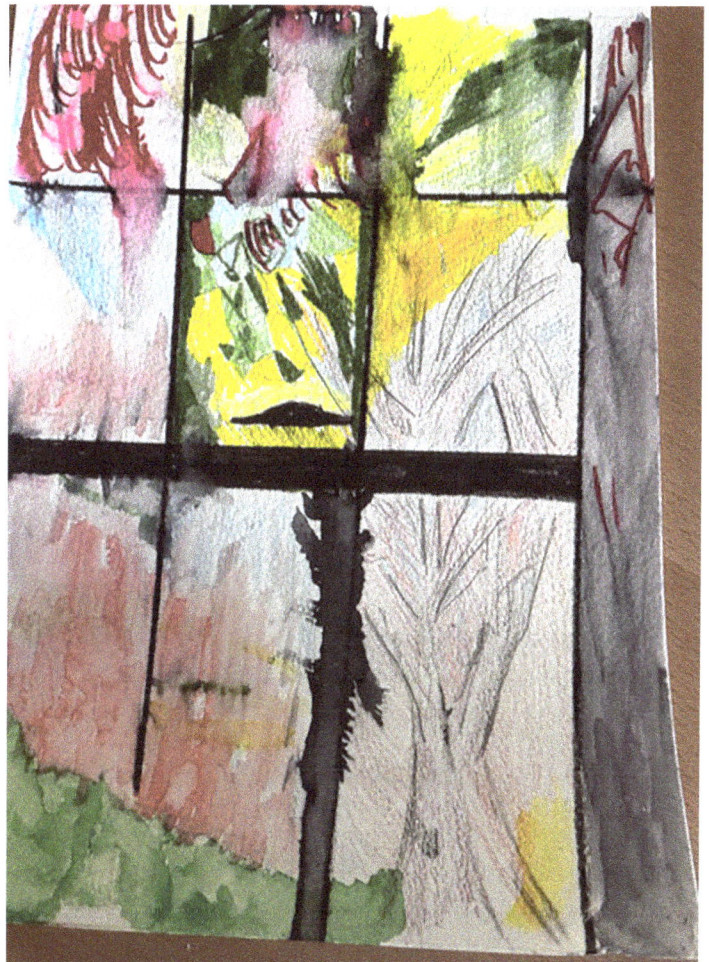

January 2021

I really do not want this post to seem maudlin. My record for dementia sleep is 20 hours over one day. The dreams were more fun than regular life. LOL PS: Nursing home staff often disparage this sleep, figuring nothing is going on in our dementia heads. Excuse me, but maybe you just can't imagine time travels joy. Jealous . . . a little?

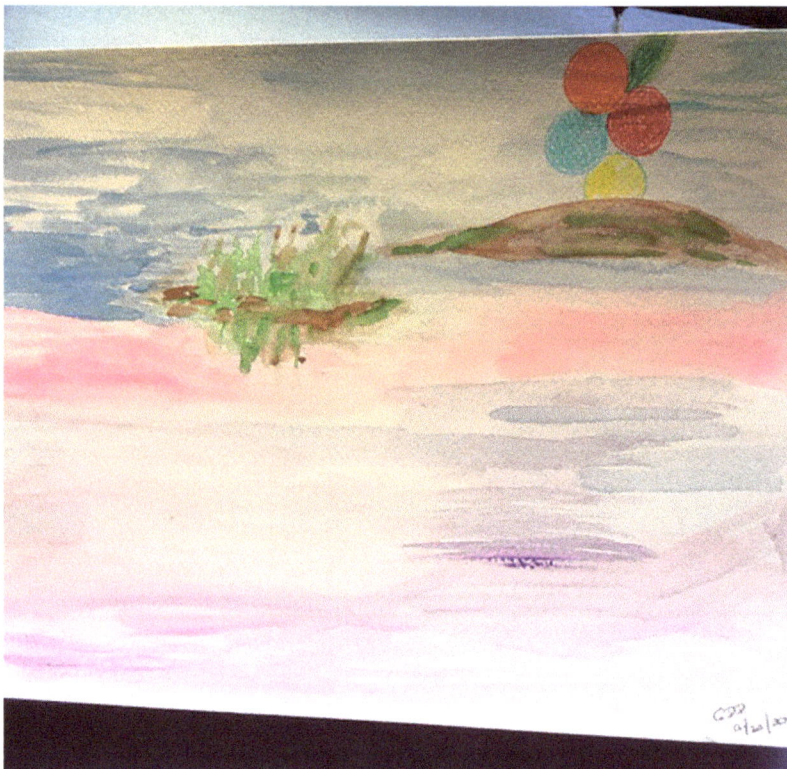

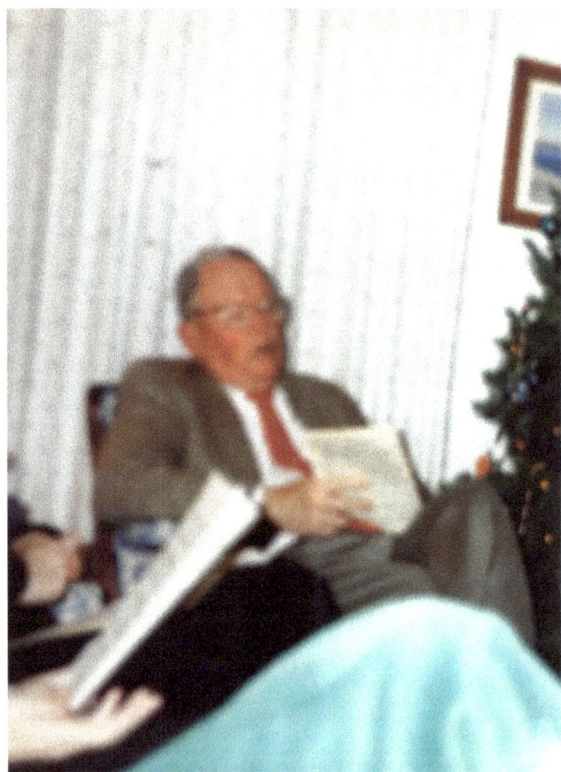

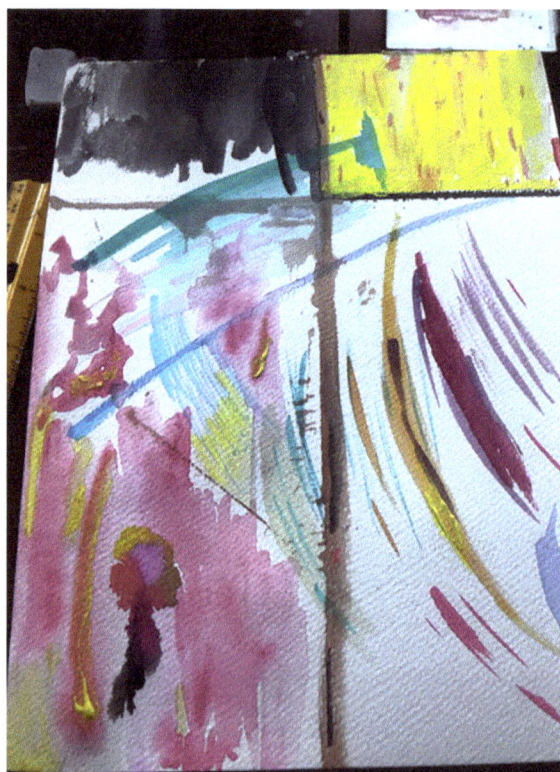

him. "Be anxious for nothing, but in *everything* by prayer and supplication, with thanksgiving, let your requests be made known to God" (Philippians

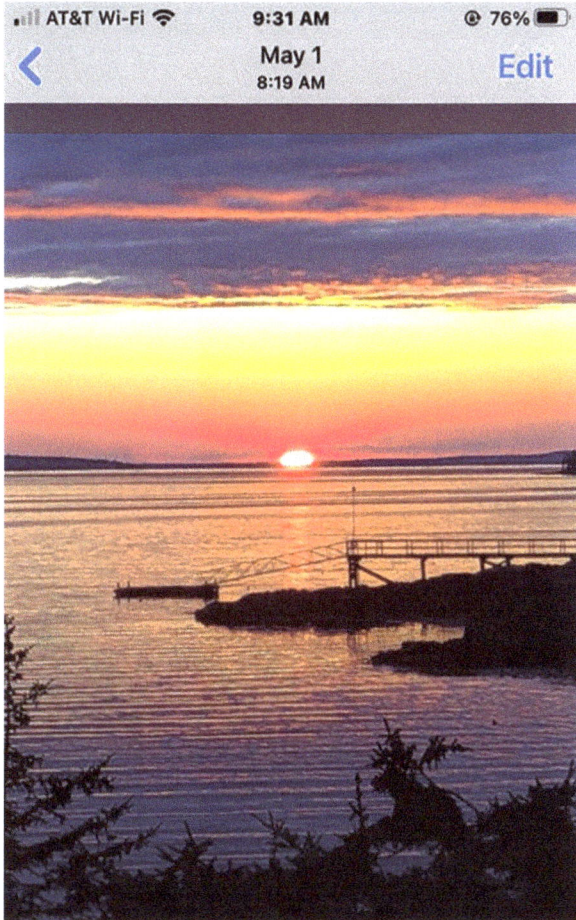

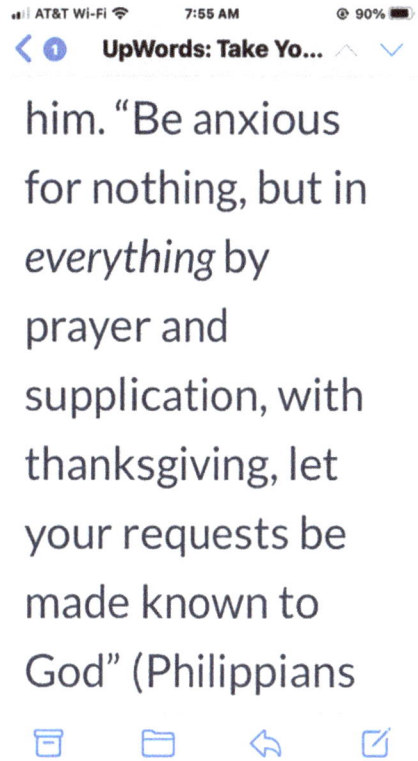

Aducanumab is the first new Alzheimer's treatment in 18 years and the first to attack the disease process. But some prominent experts say there's not enough evidence it can address cognitive symptoms.

February 2021

I have discovered a new symptom that I will call instant dementia. The thought is unretrievable immediately, like less than a second. It was confirmed when I woke up from the nap with two eye coverings on. LOL

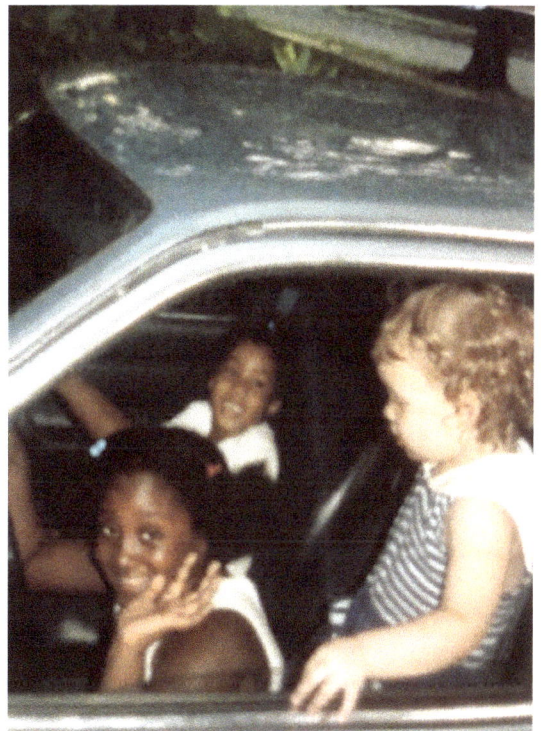

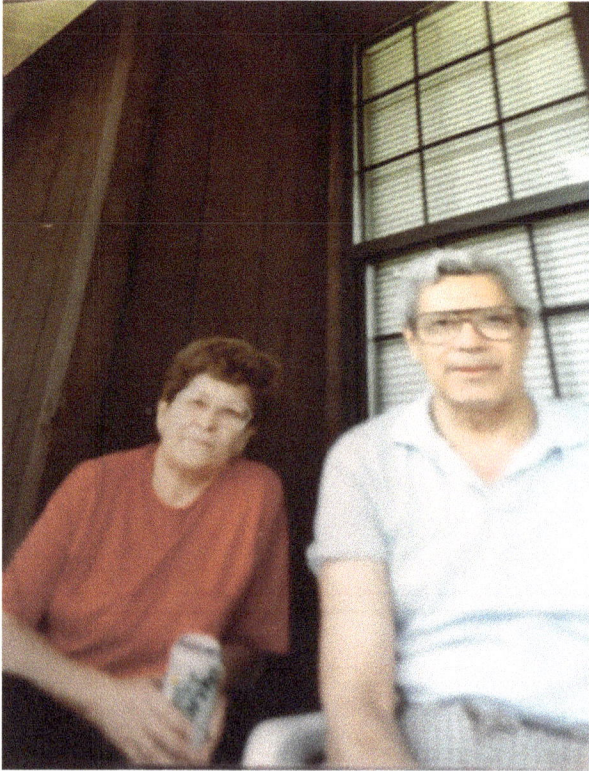

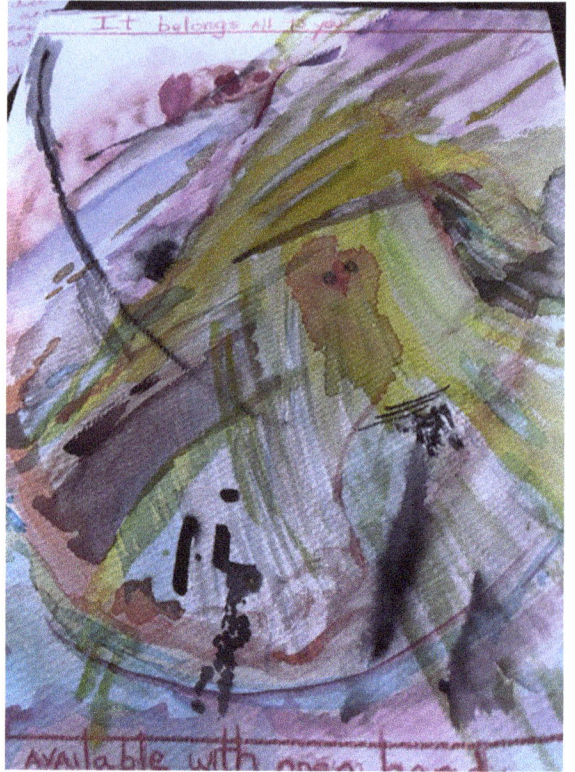

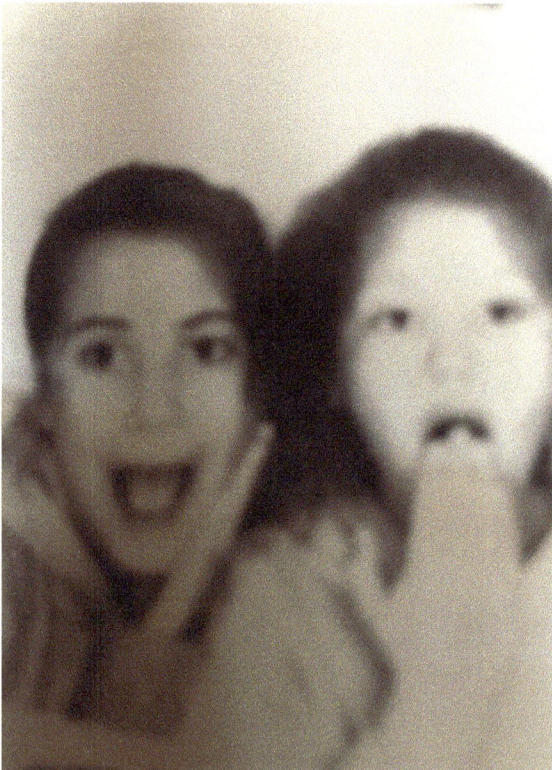

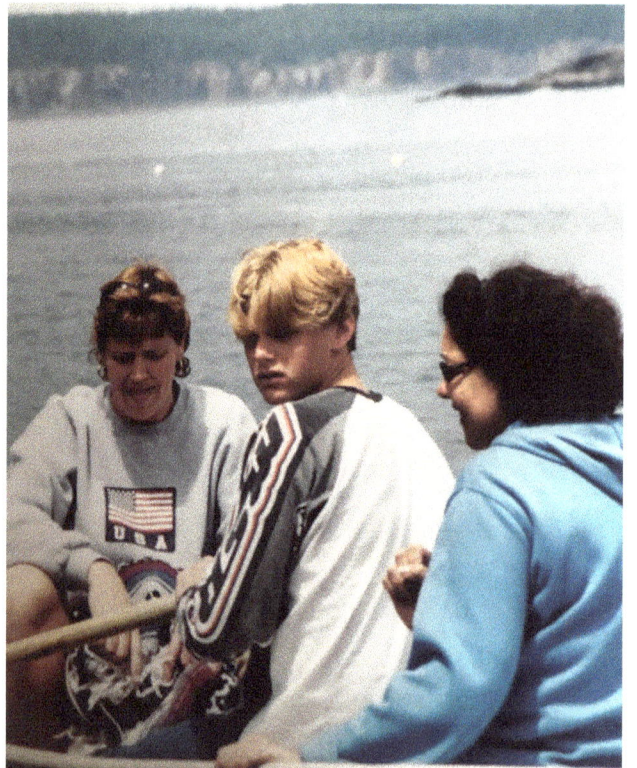

June 2021

I guess this dementia dude ought to have figured, but I recently became aware that regular people are disquieted when we have our more regular-person moments of acuity. Concerning, really. A sign perhaps that the caregiving is suspect.

May 2021

Dementia is learning to dance in the rain. The problem with the regular people who dominate the dementia community is that they are afraid to take a twirl or two with us. True?

May 2021

We dementia dudes and dudettes really have to learn to be at peace with confusion. Or learn to enjoy it, like . . . I forgot.

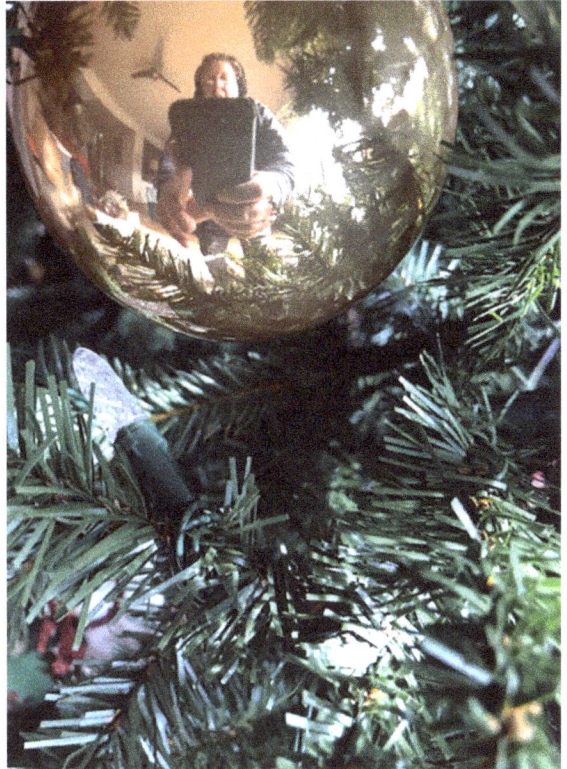

Don't dare call it denial when people choose to live fully with dementia. Call it courage, call it optimism, call it defiance or just call it living.
#EndStigma

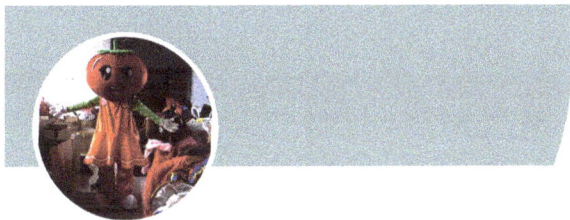

@LEAD_Coalition

Dallas Dixon
Dementia author and wanna be dementia advocate and activist.
Trenton, New Jersey, United States · Contact info
500+ connections

Open to   Add section   More

I am a tomato
Princeton University

February 2021
Pretty cool.

Don't dare call it denial when people choose to live fully with dementia. Call it courage, call it optimism, call it defiance or just call it living.

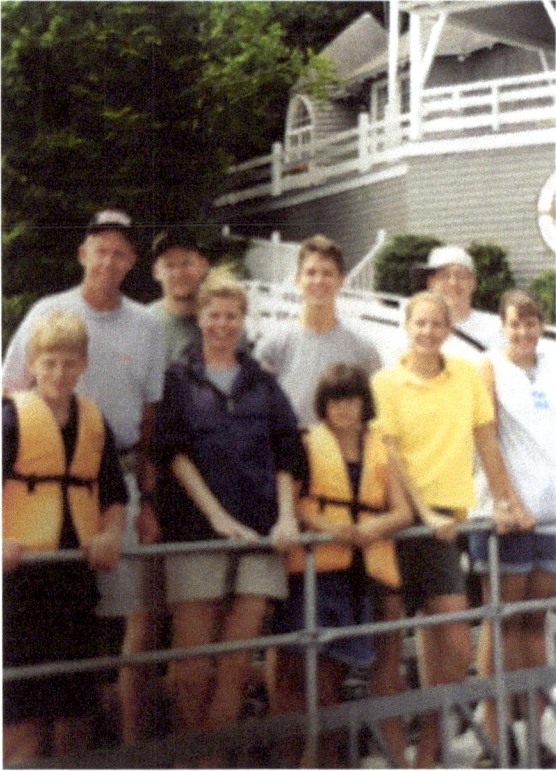

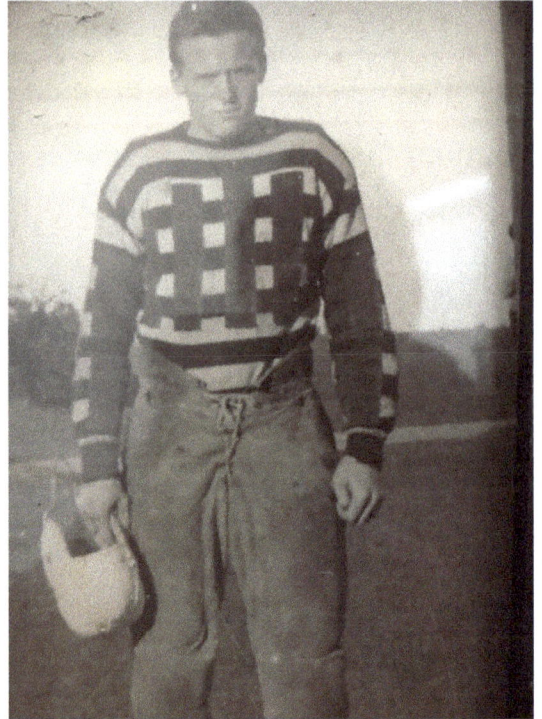

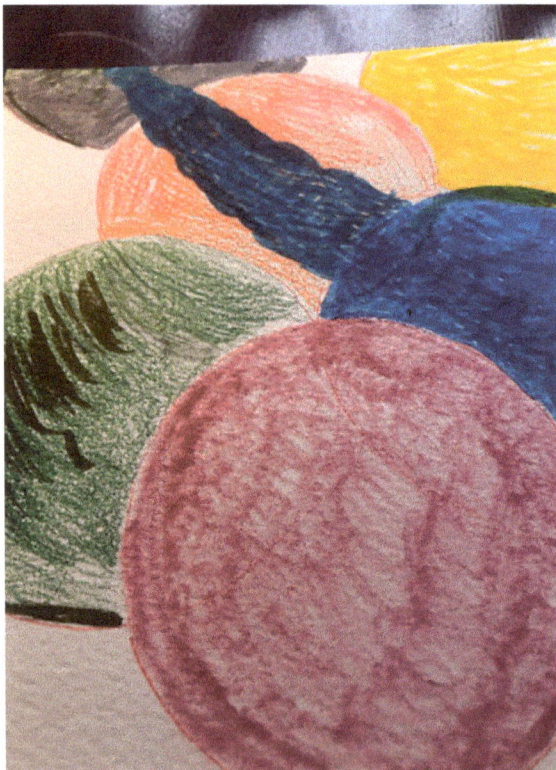

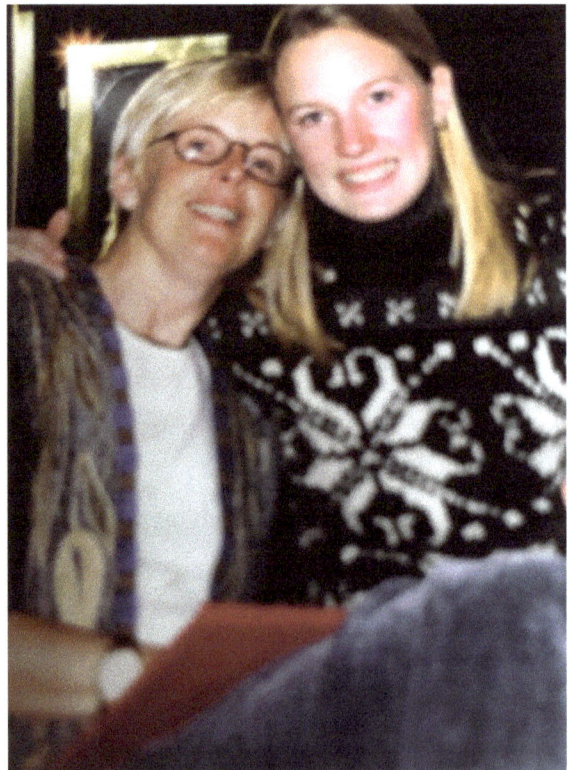

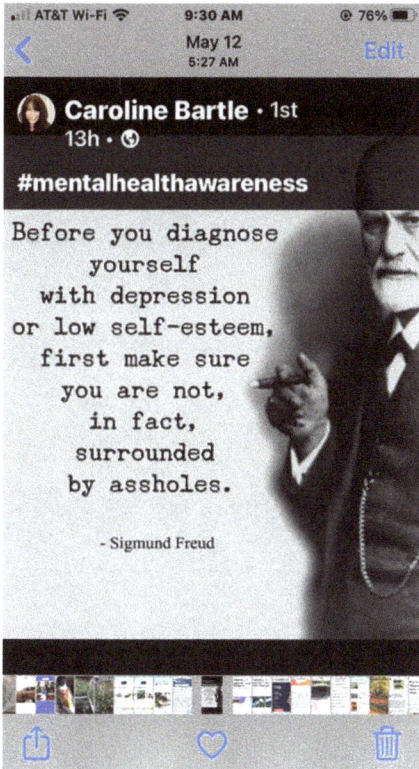

Caroline Bartle · 1st
13h · 🌐

#mentalhealthawareness

Before you diagnose
yourself
with depression
or low self-esteem,
first make sure
you are not,
in fact,
surrounded
by assholes.

- Sigmund Freud

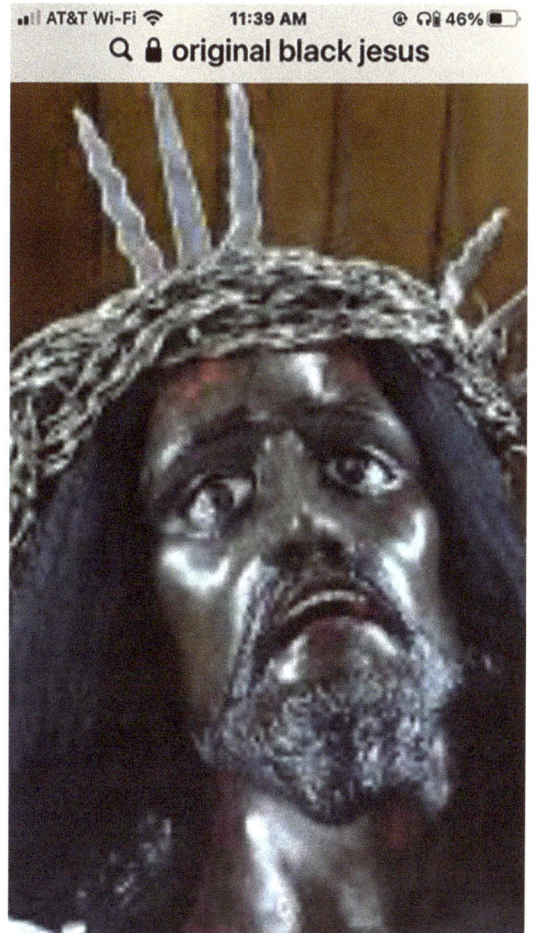

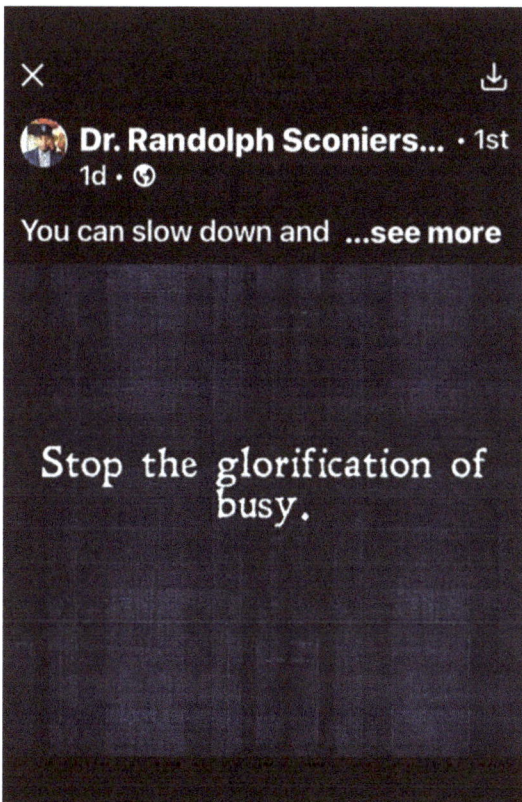

✕   ⬇

Dr. Randolph Sconiers... · 1st
1d · 🌐

You can slow down and ...see more

Stop the glorification of
busy.

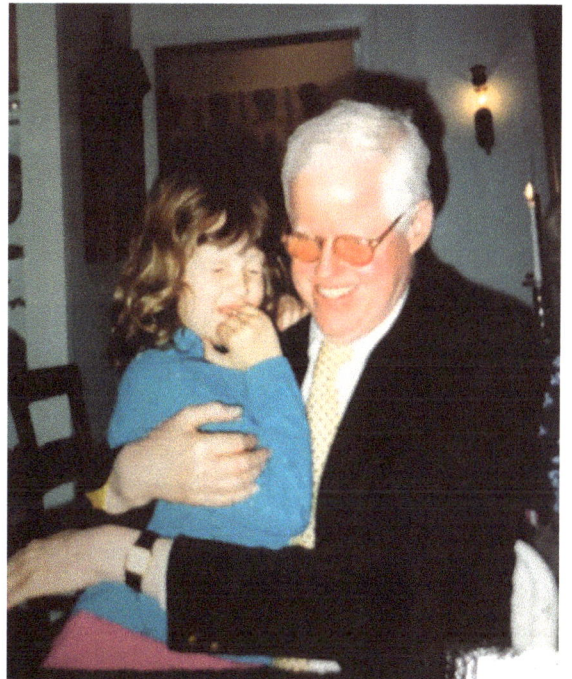

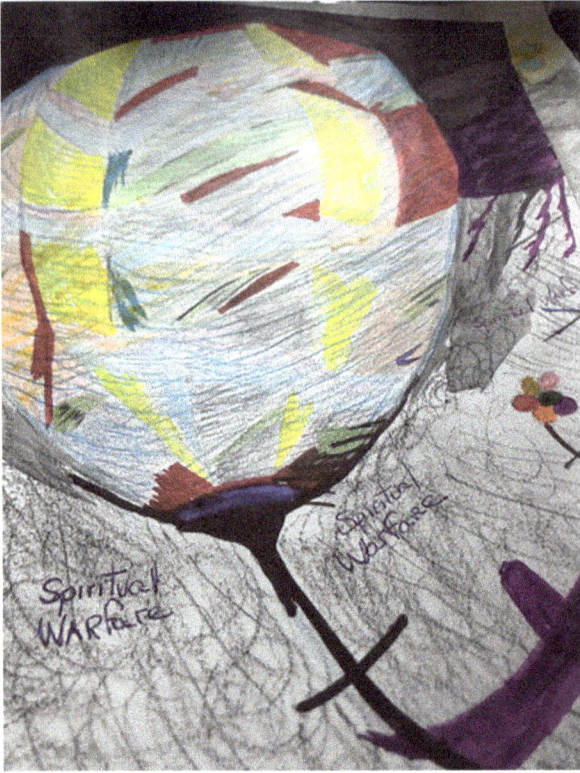

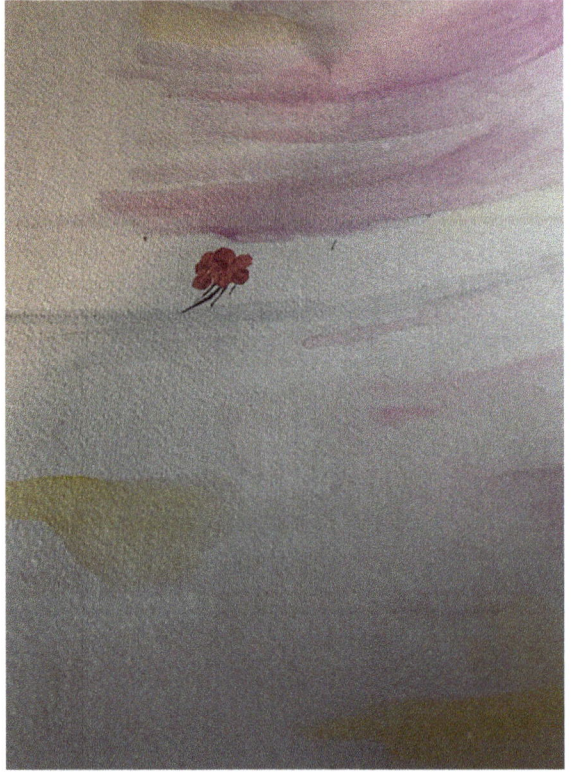

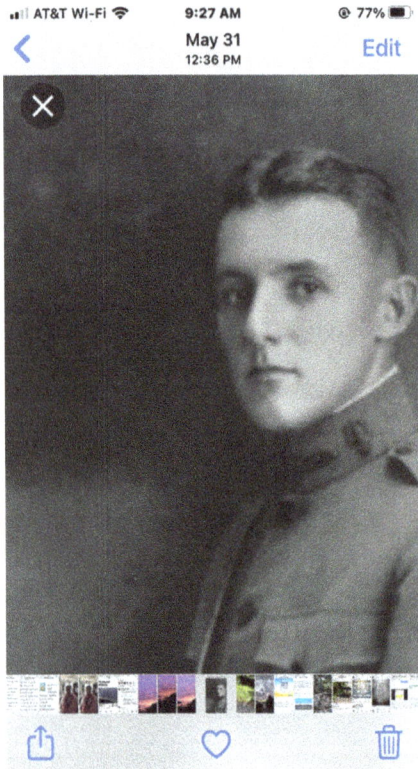

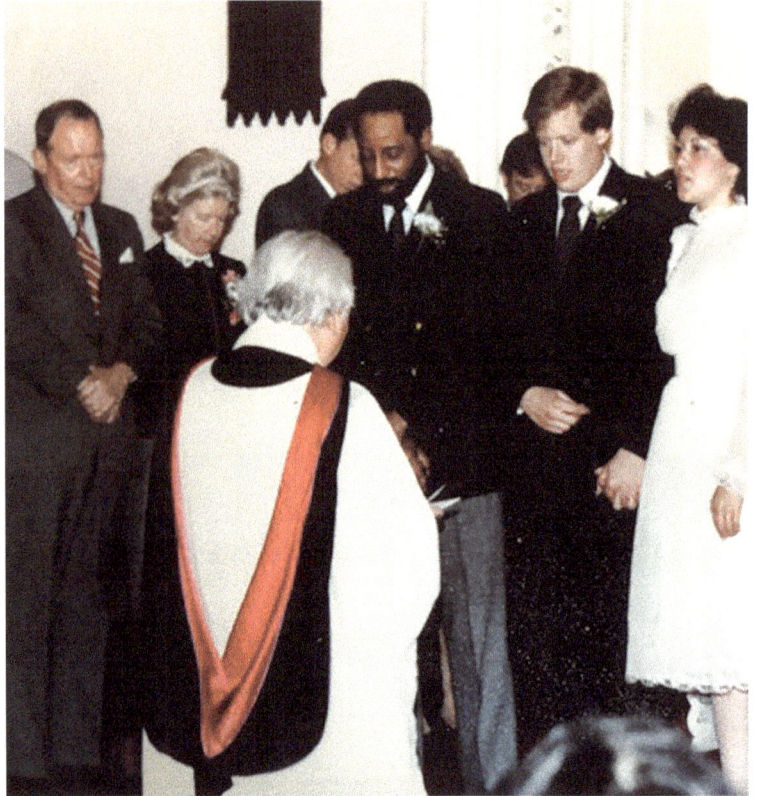

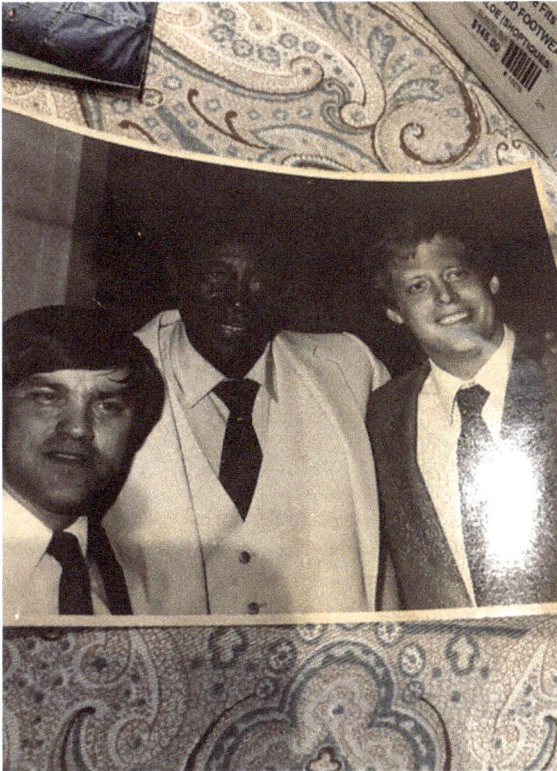

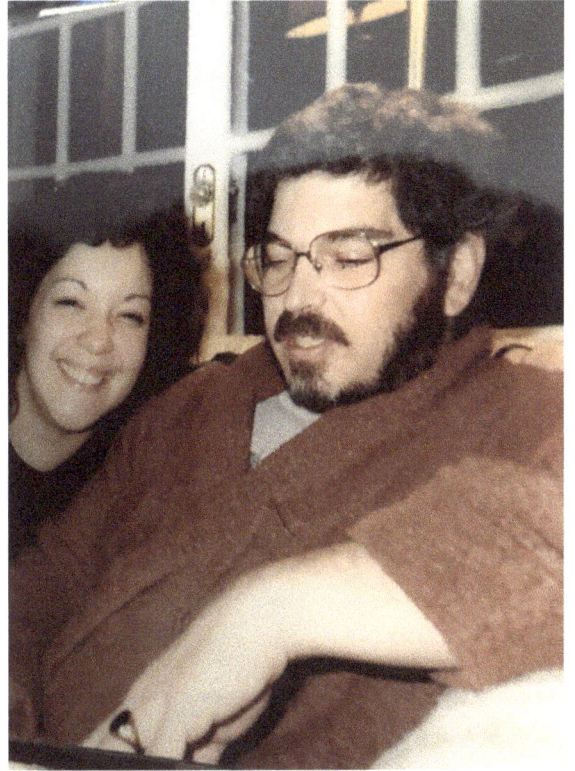

September 2020

If you are in the dementia world and you can't find joy, you've got work to do.

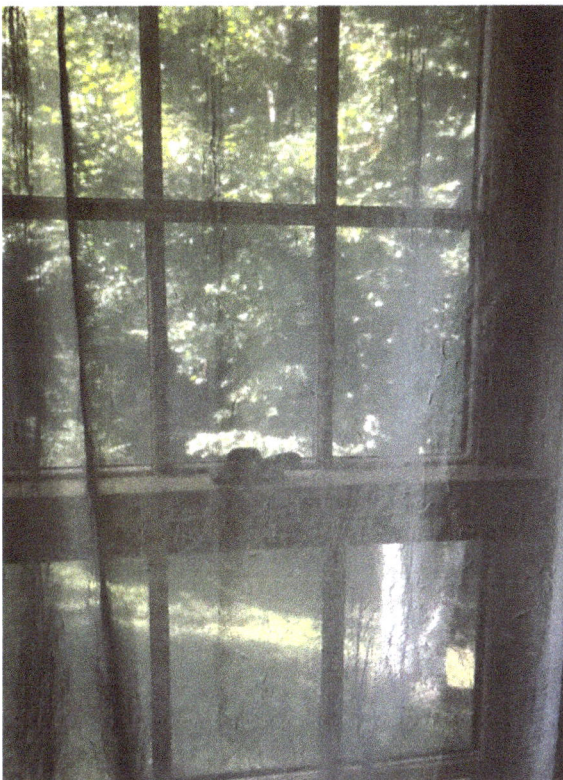

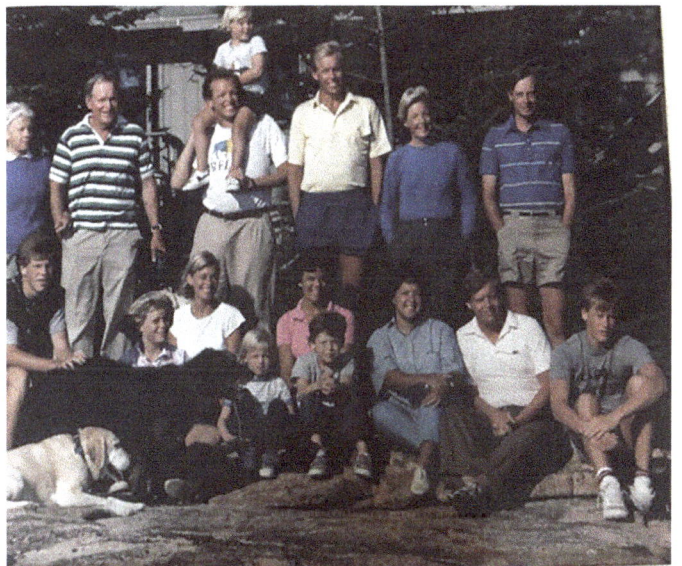

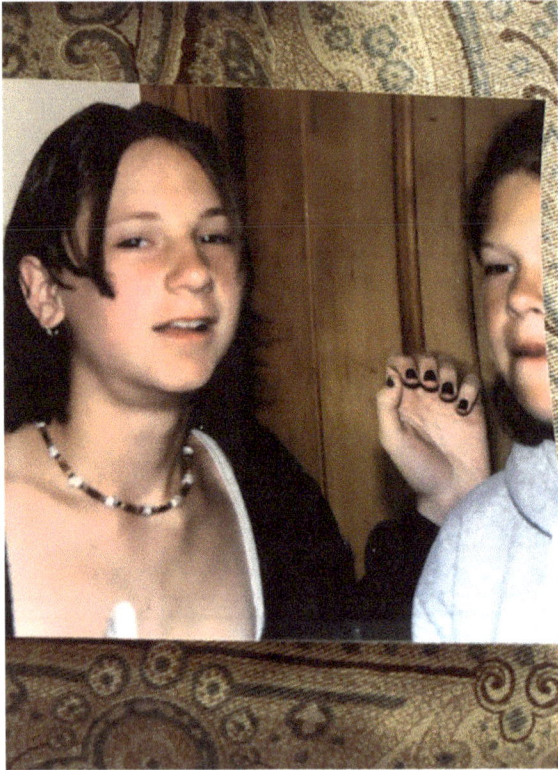
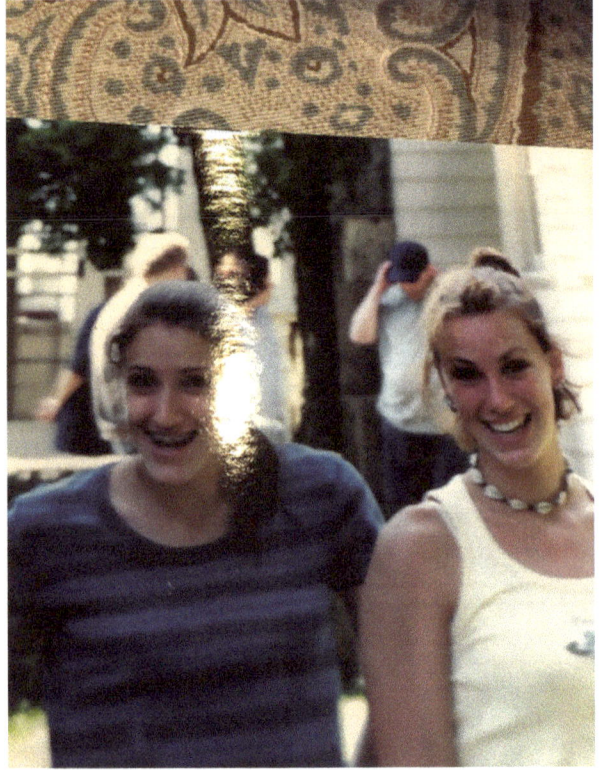
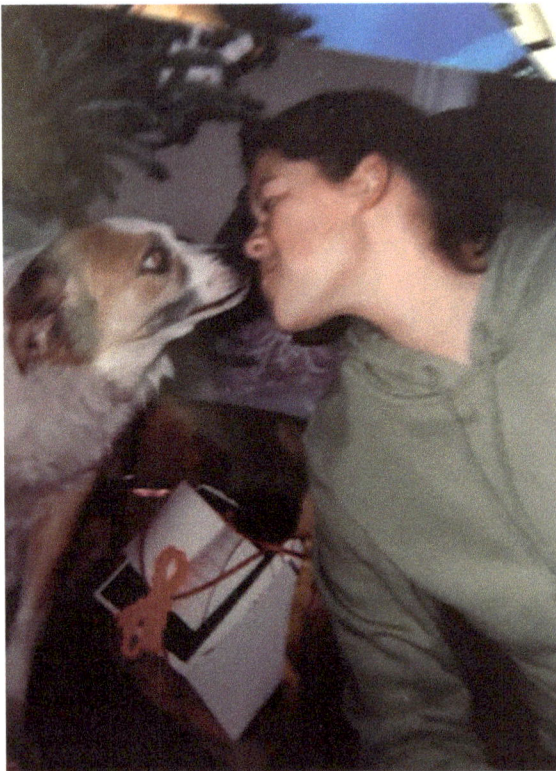
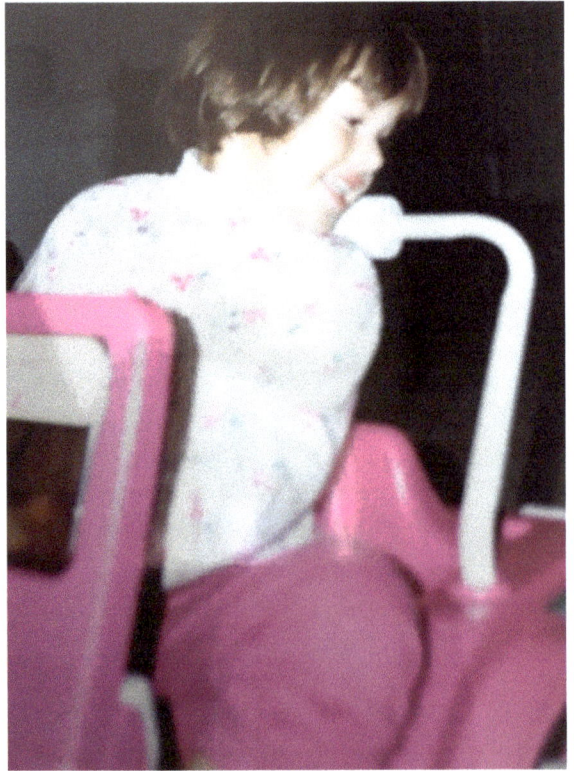

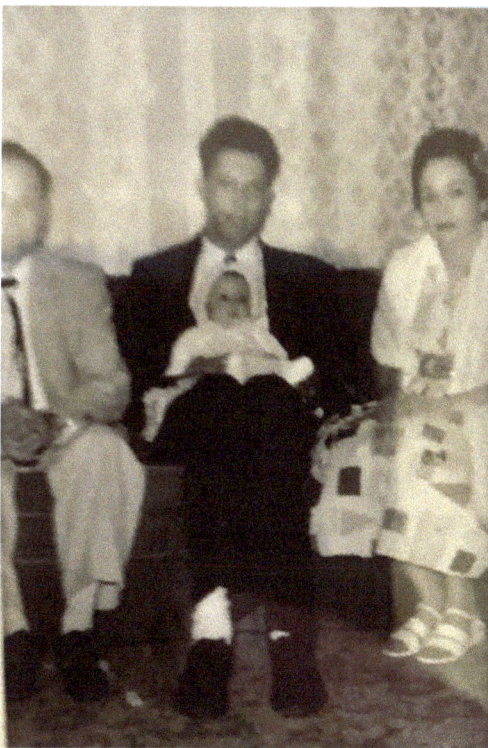

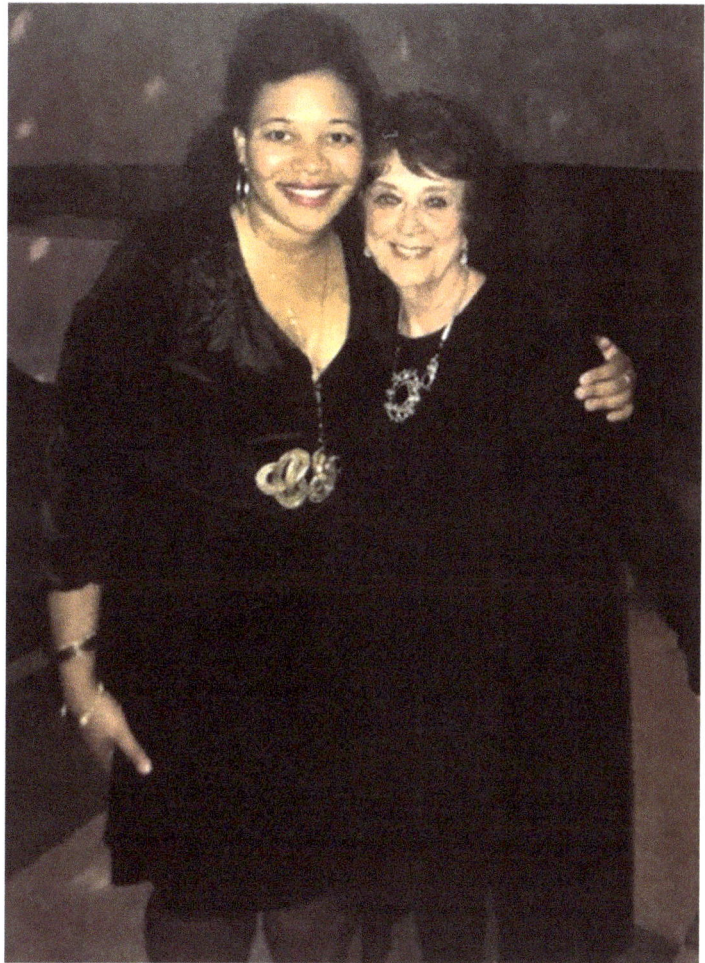

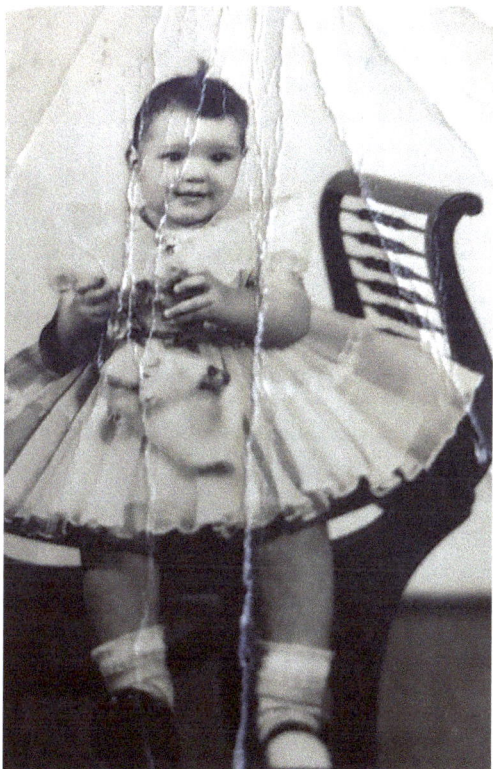

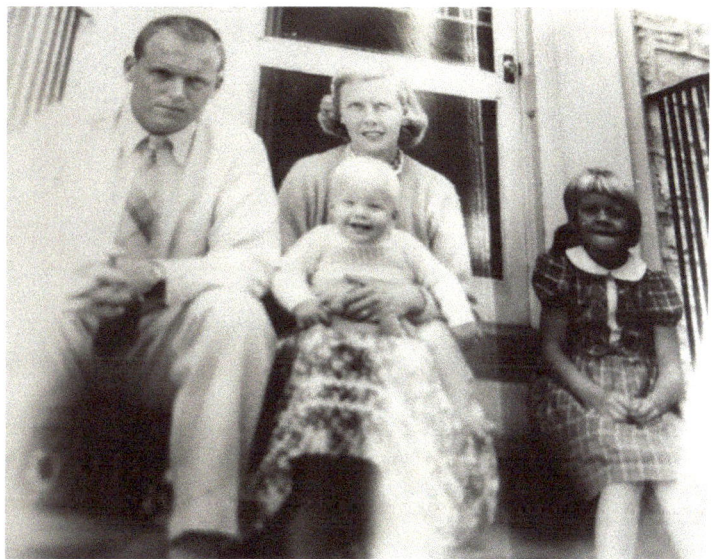

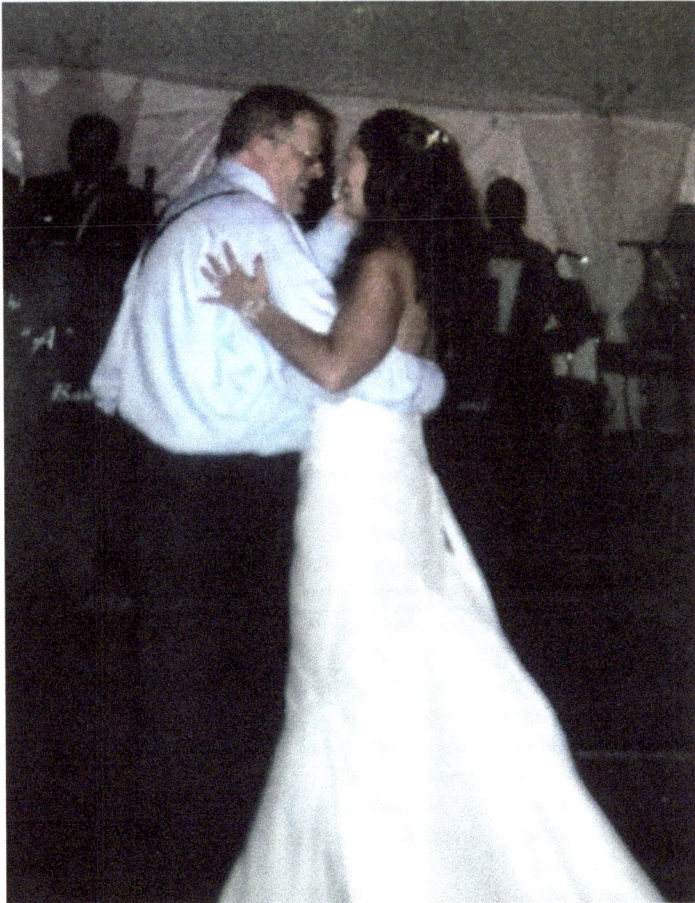
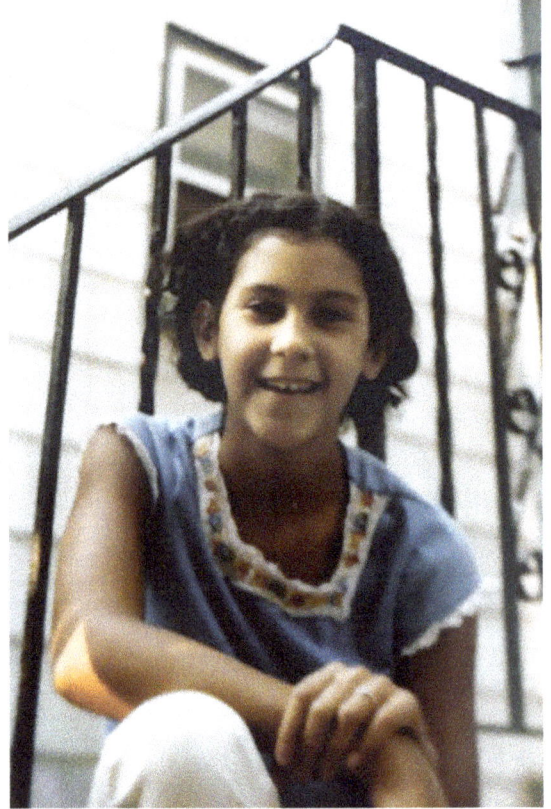
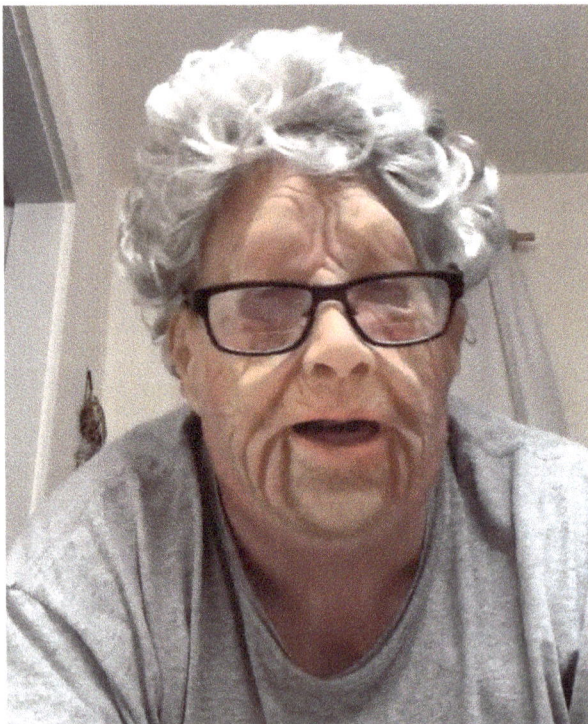
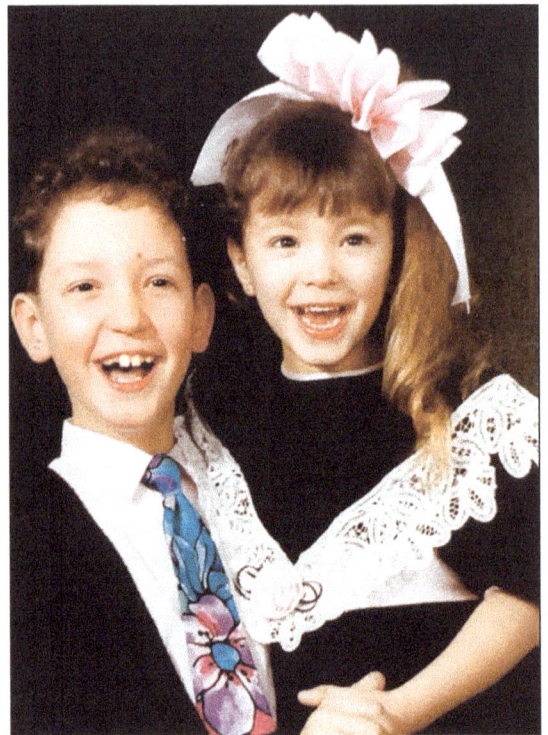

34:39

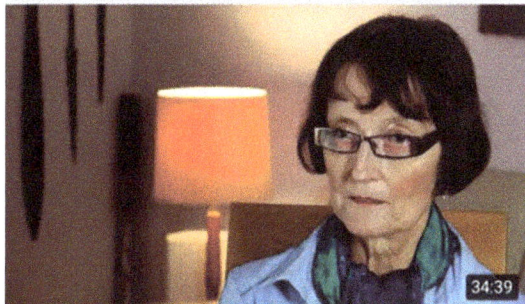

Christine Bryden: A conversation about dementia

Aged Care Quality and Safety Commission · 13K views · 7 years ago

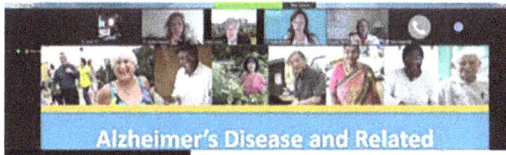

Alzheimer's Disease and Related

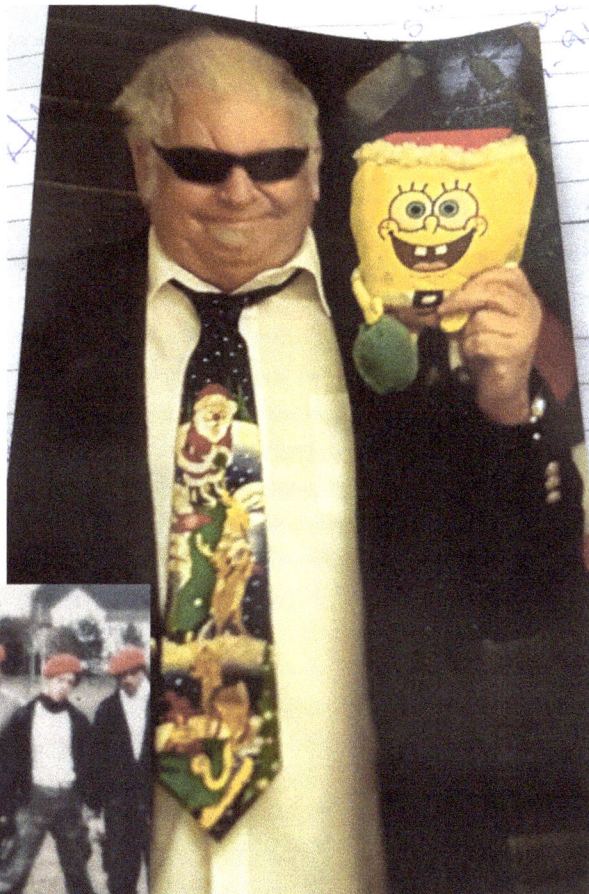

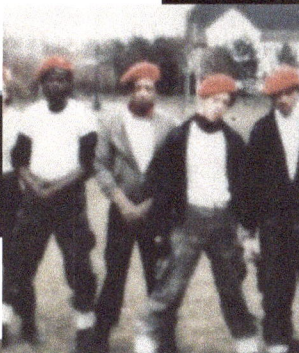

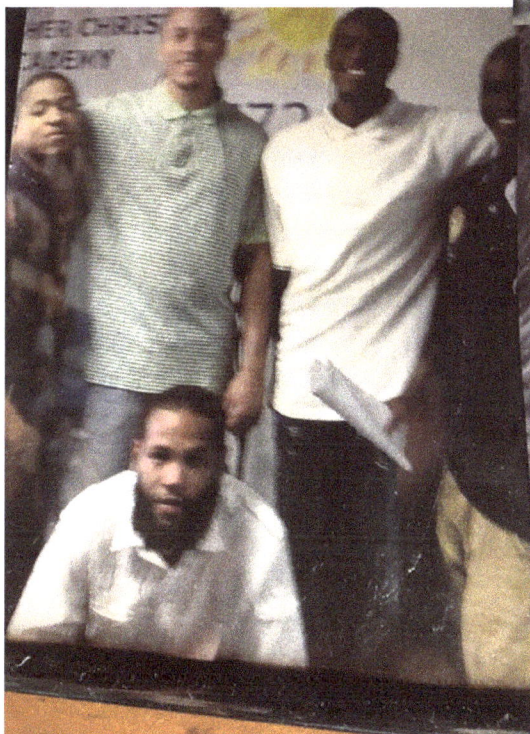

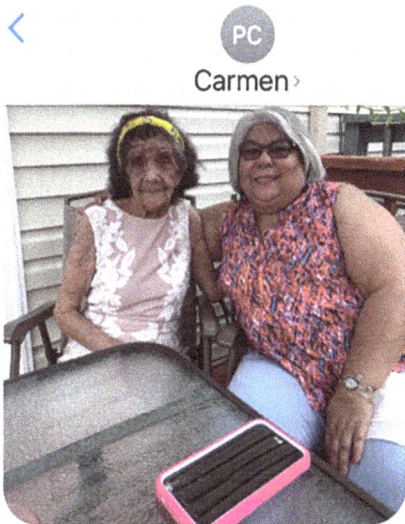

Here's mom
with her niece,

67

🍀 MARY BARDIN 🍀 • 1st
Operations Manager at The Alzheimer Society of Ireland
1d

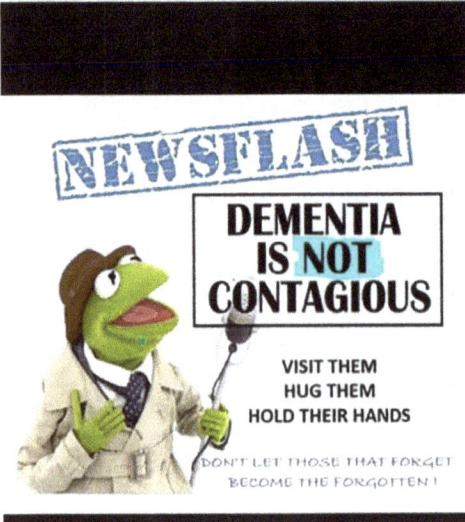

NEWSFLASH

DEMENTIA IS NOT CONTAGIOUS

VISIT THEM
HUG THEM
HOLD THEIR HANDS

DON'T LET THOSE THAT FORGET BECOME THE FORGOTTEN!

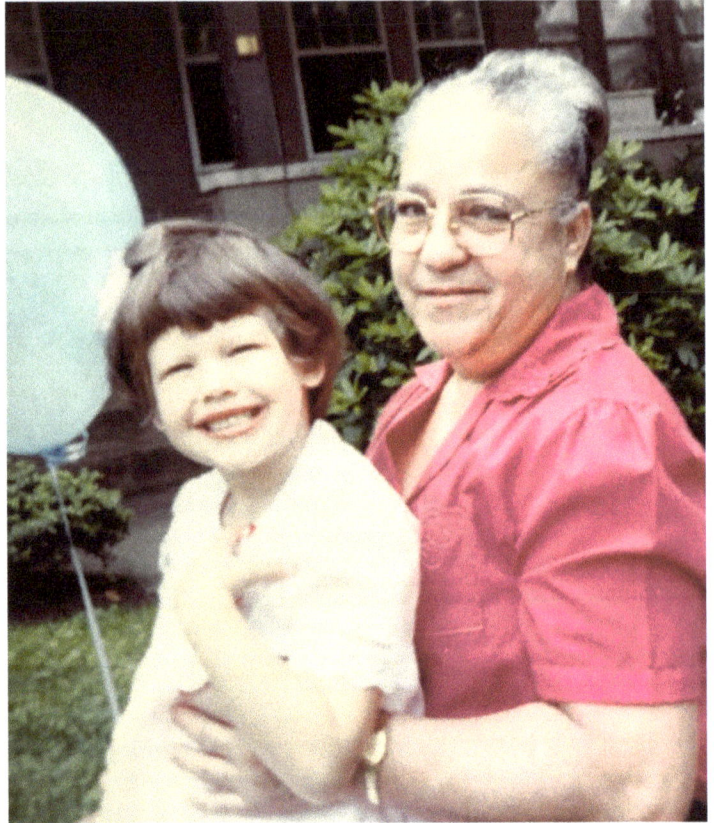

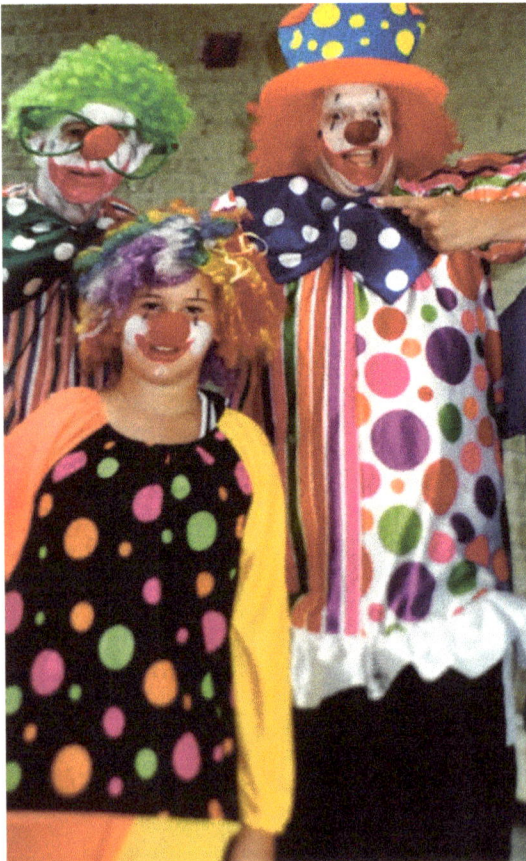

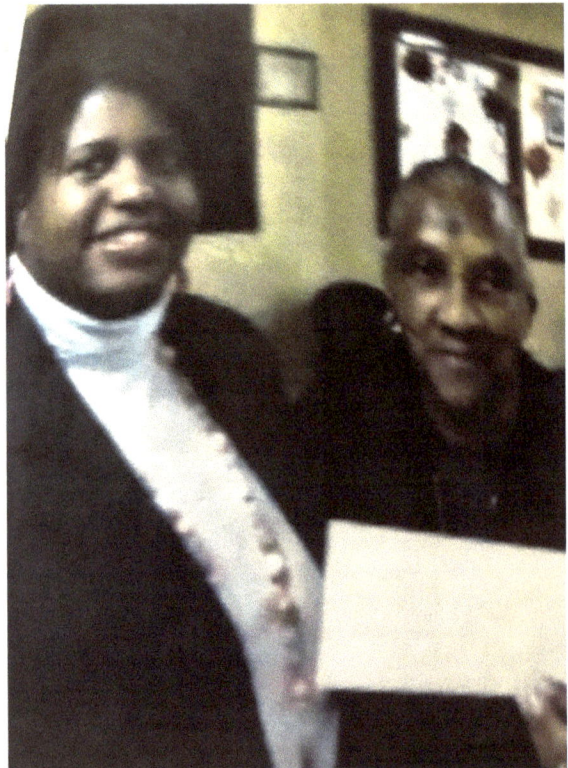

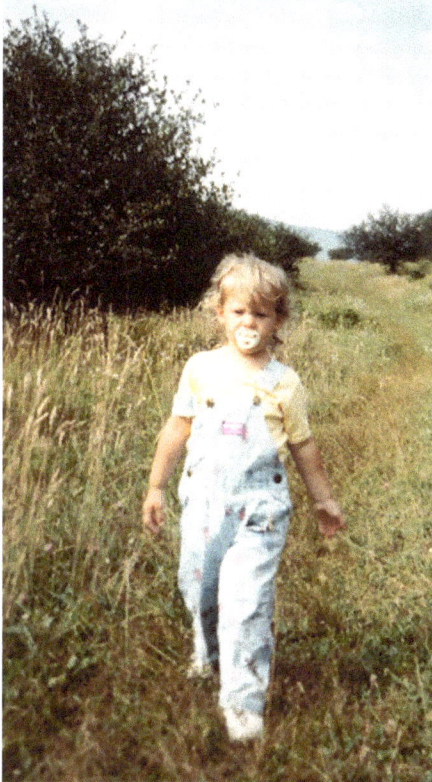

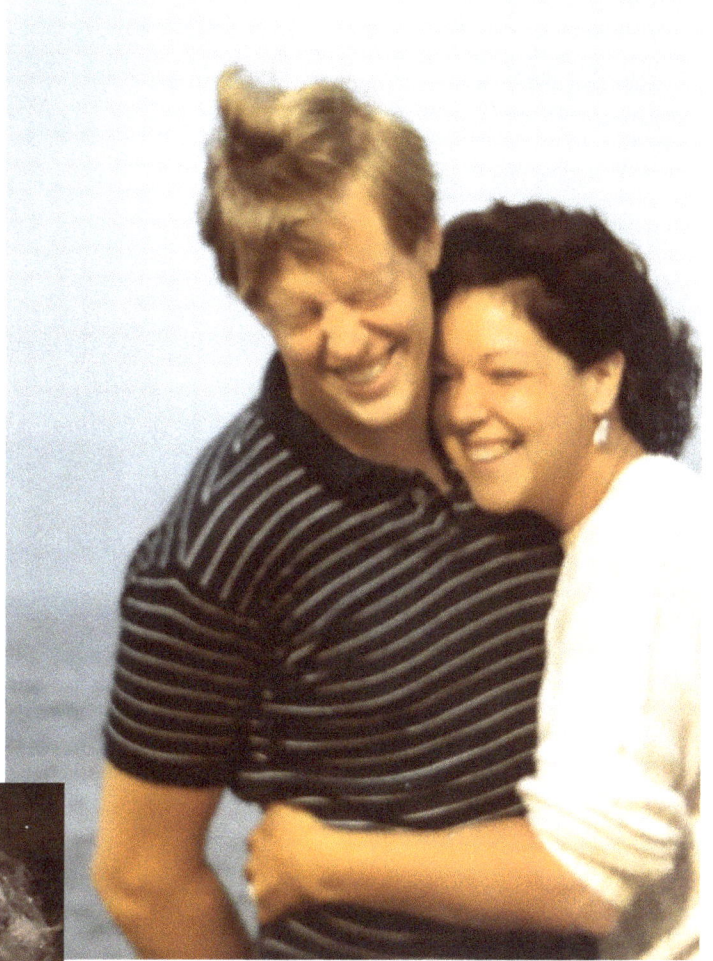

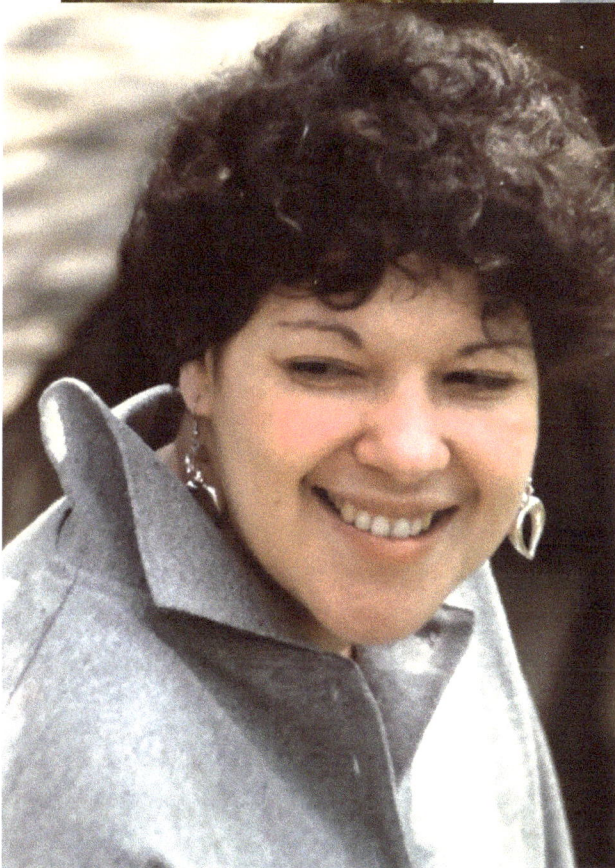

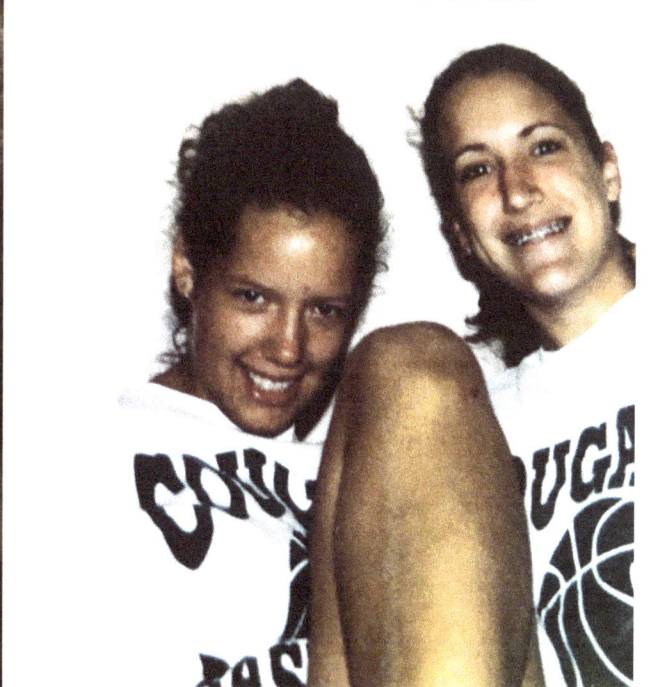

integrity of elections.
What Arizona's
Republican senators
arranged, by contrast,
is what you'd get if you
crossed a clown
pageant with a QAnon
convention and made
the whole thing open
bar. The whole mess
would be entertaining
if it weren't so
destructive.

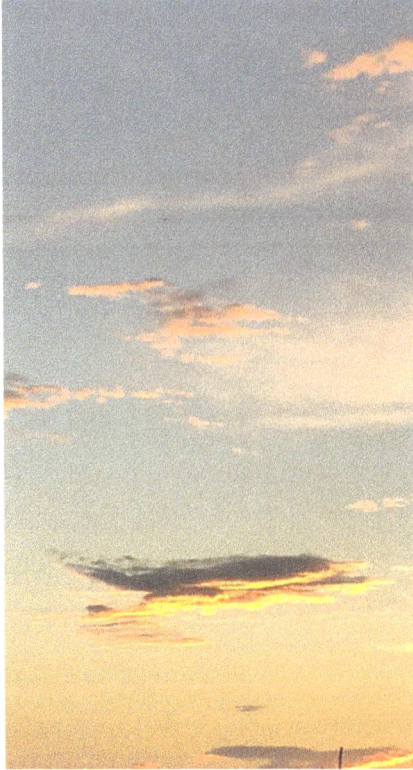

Where G.O.P. efforts like

Post time is 6:47 p.m.
Eastern time on Saturday.

Breathing Through the Rectum Saves Oxygen-Starved Mice and Pigs

Japanese scientists who
studied an unusual
method of delivering
oxygen in mammals hope
to one day try it in people.

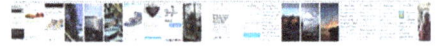

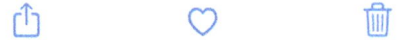

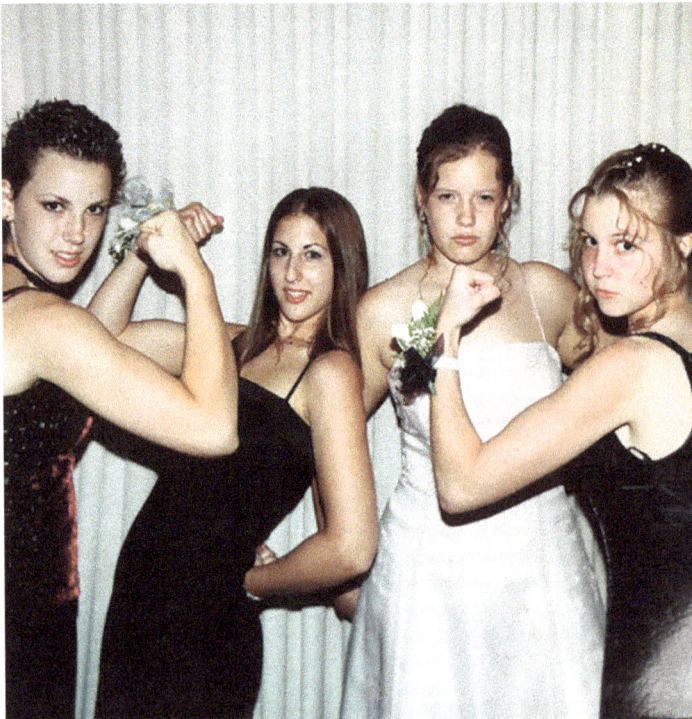

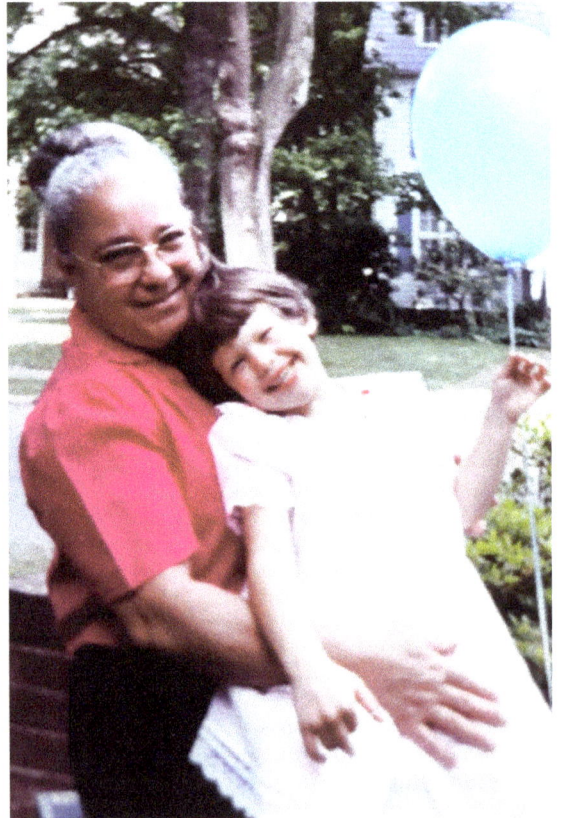

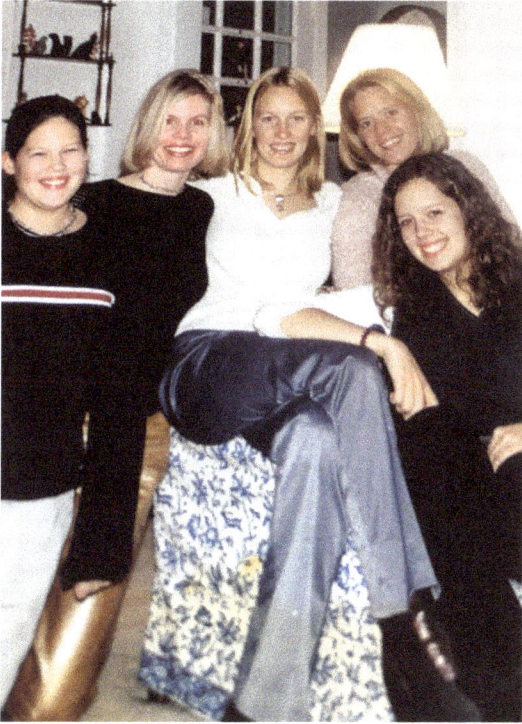
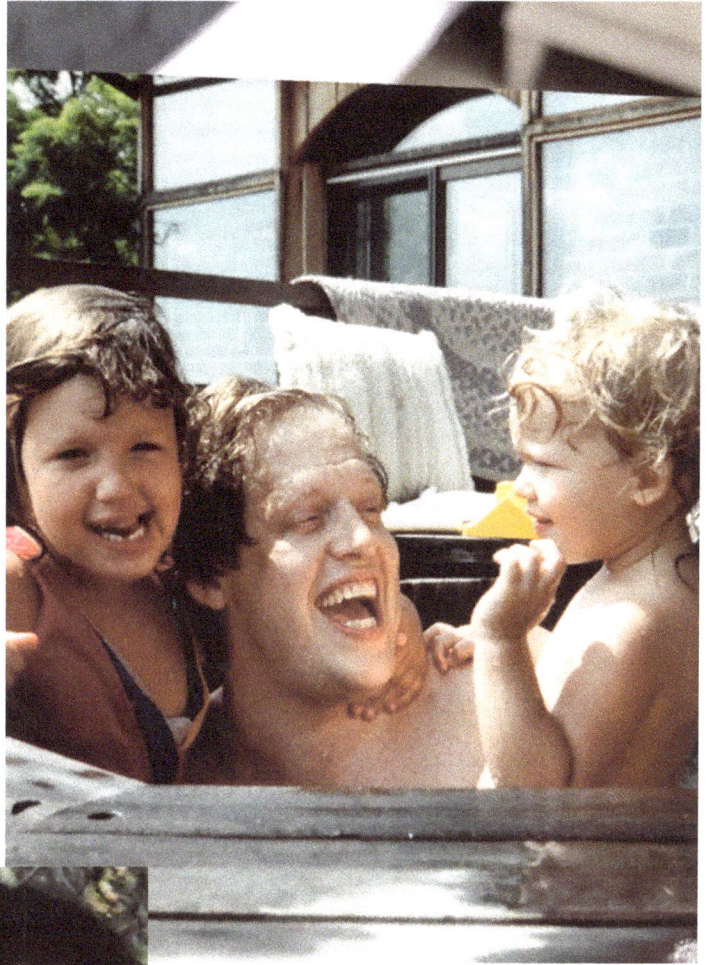
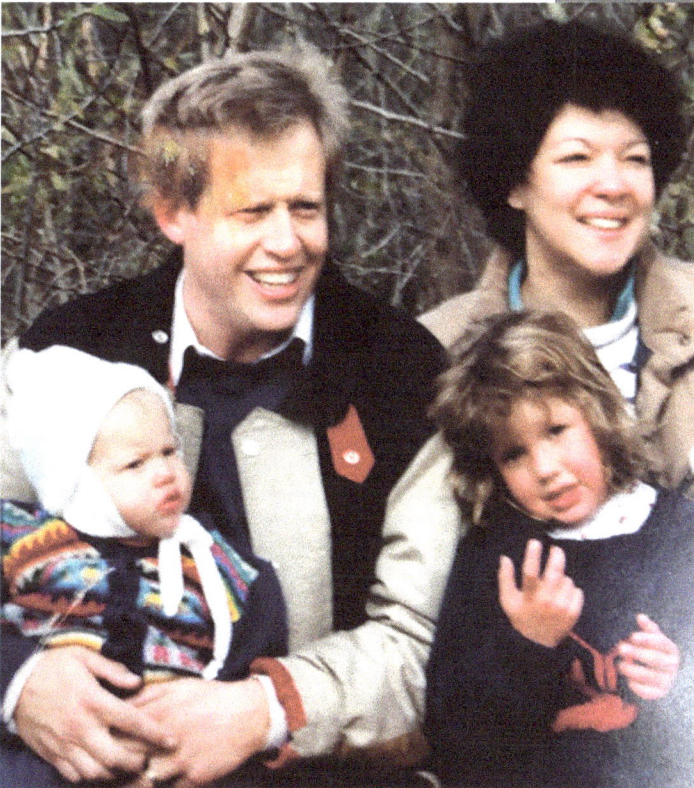
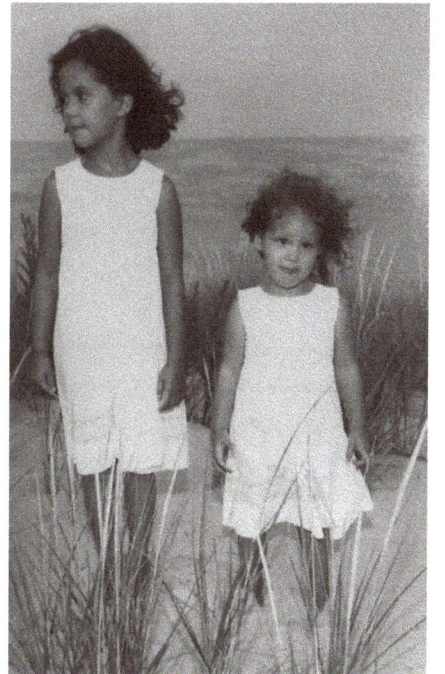

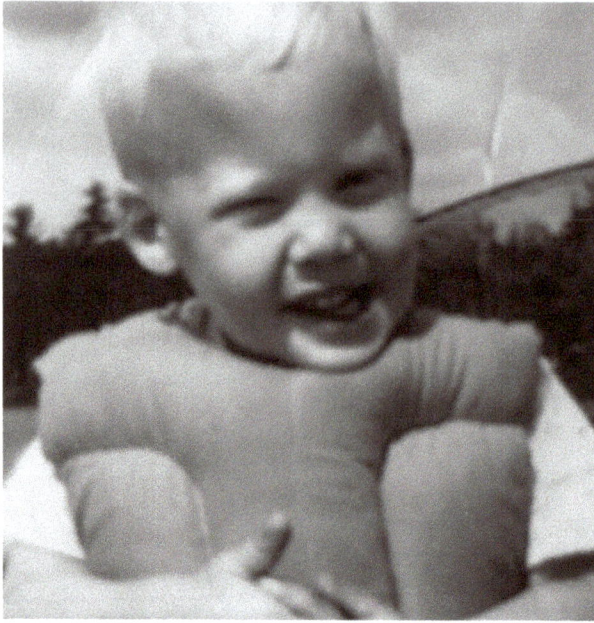

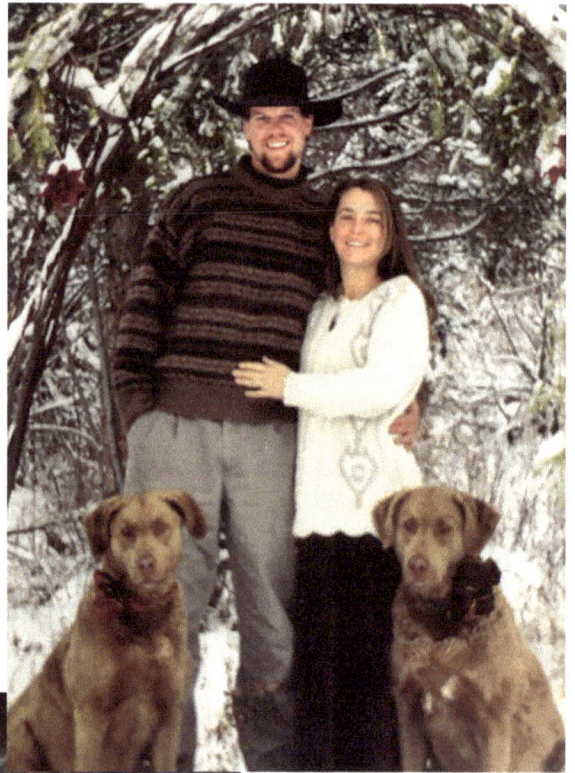

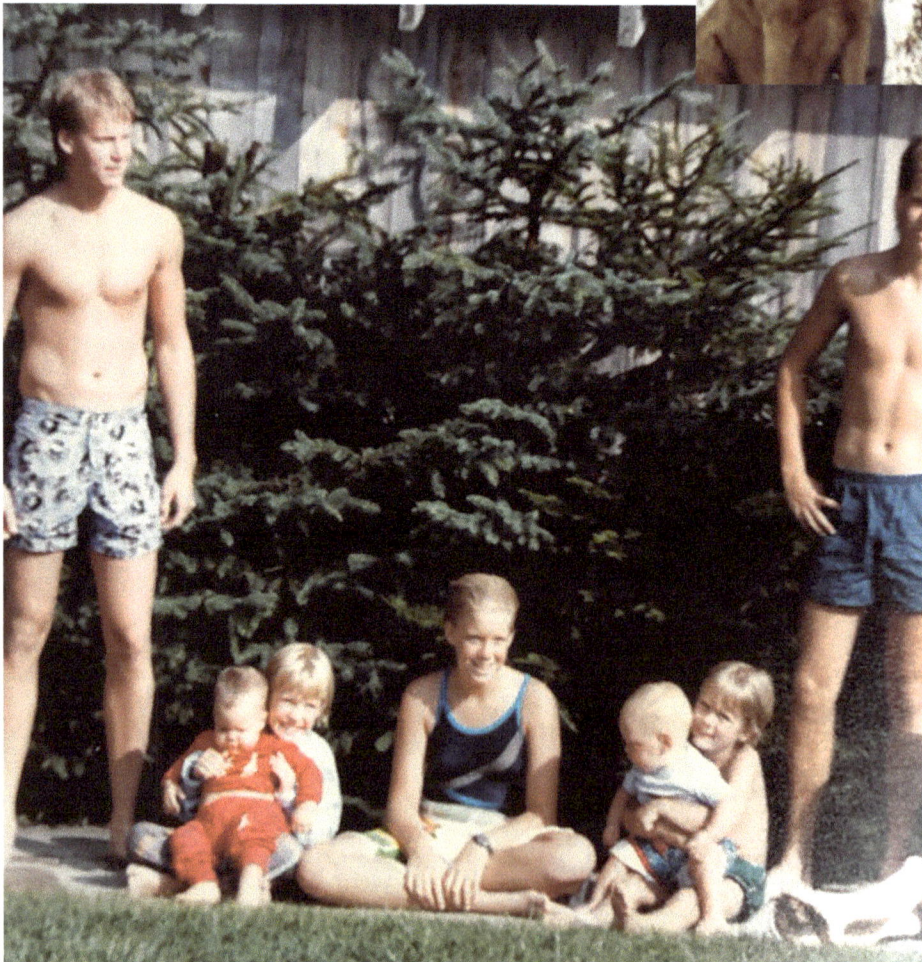

Give God power over your death experience.

We (ok I) will only mess it up trying to organize it. (Before dementia too.)

When u gotta sleep,
you gotta sleep.
One of our all-time
friends.

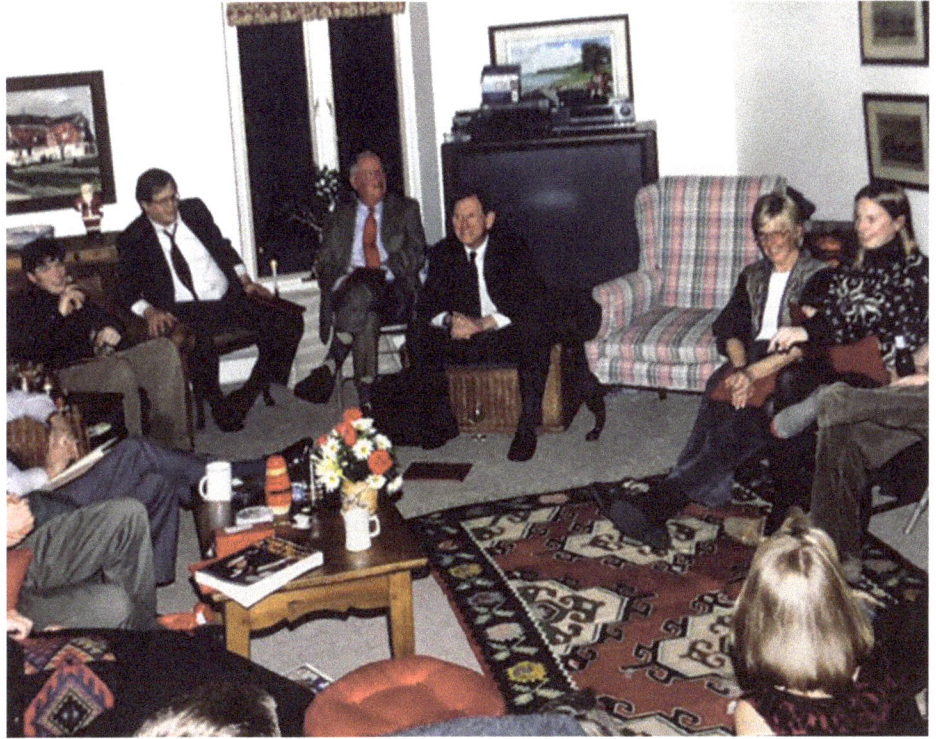

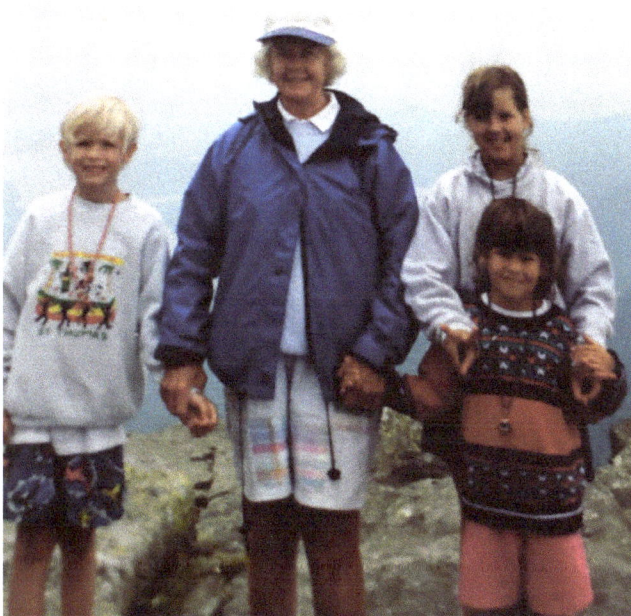

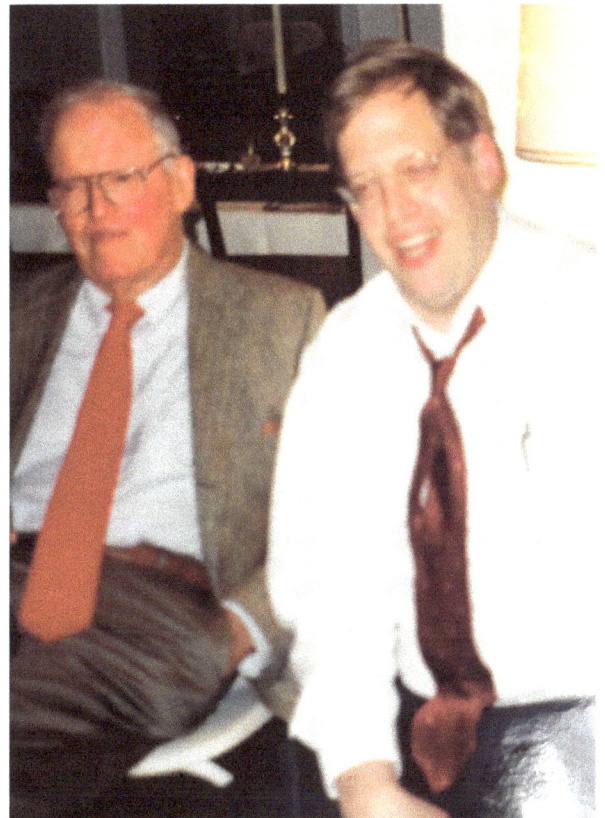

Sleeeeeeeeeep.

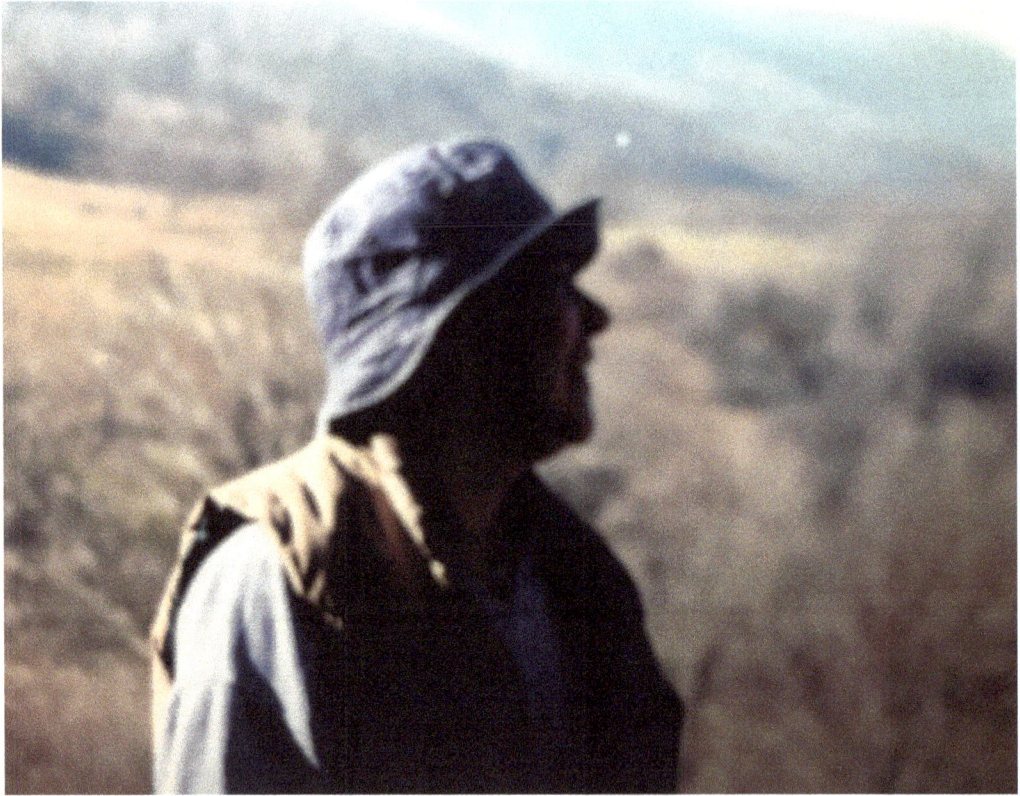

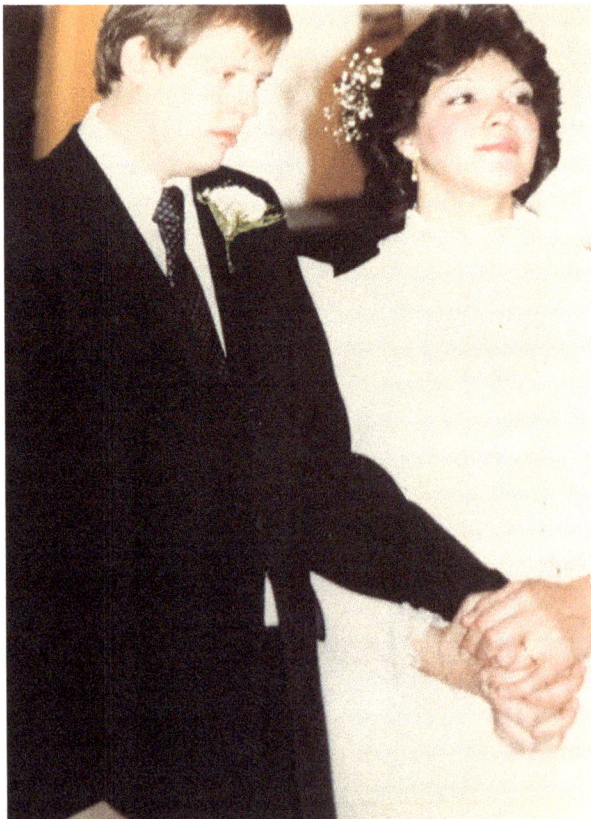

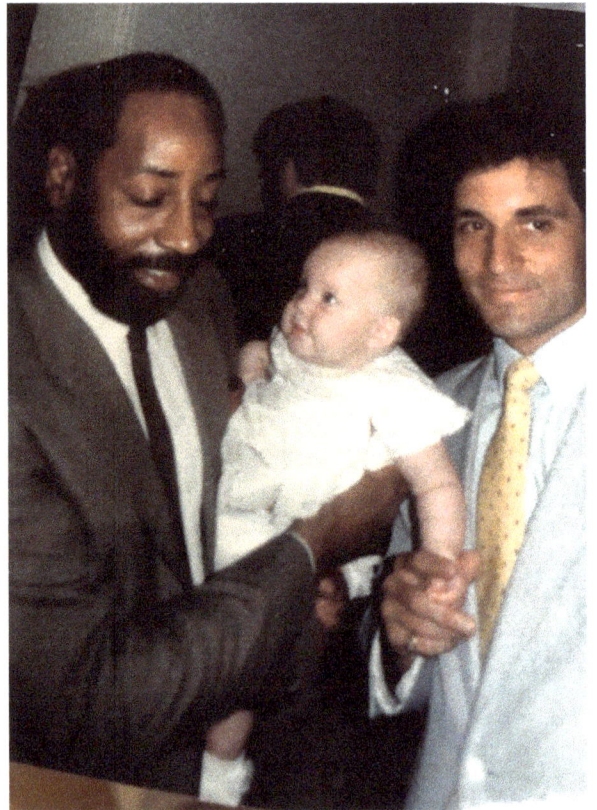

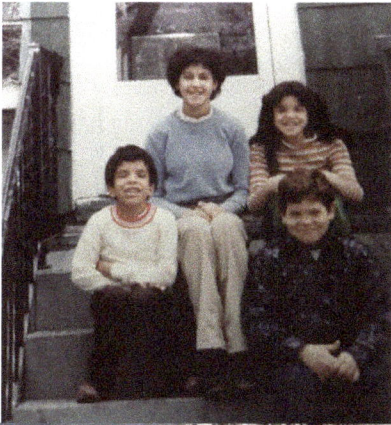

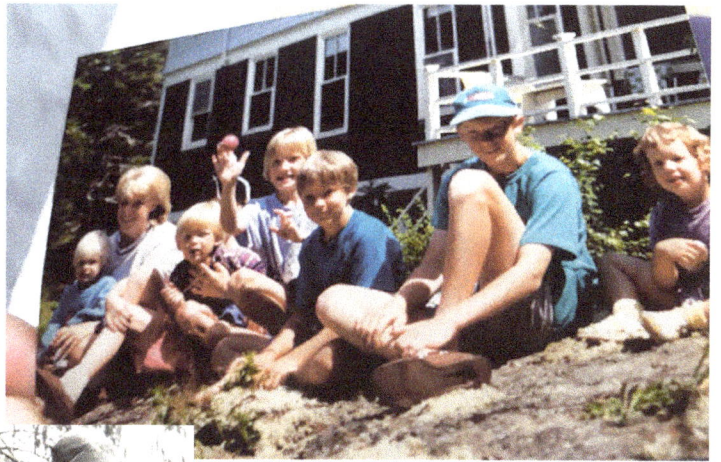

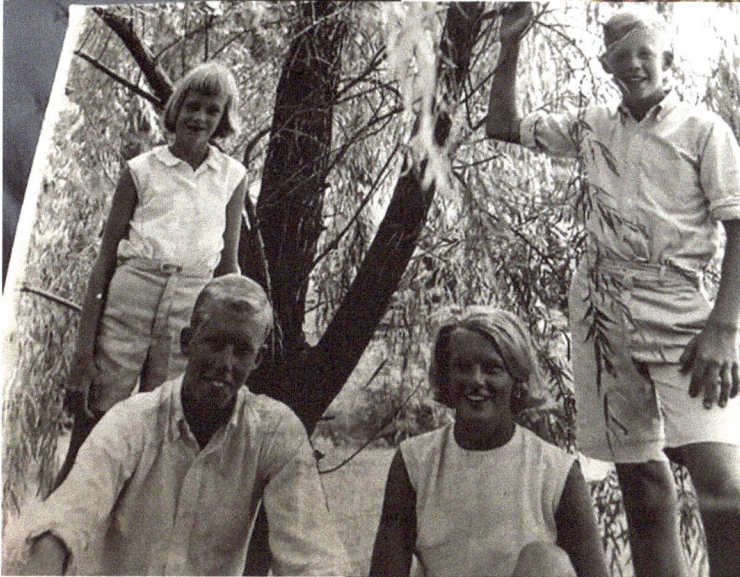

I do like dementia a lot. Even the "bad" stuff is cool.
My first hallucination: bubbles.
The dropsies: relinquishing my title of best hands in the family. The burden of greatness is lifted. Left behind in family travel: my family has learned about dementia for me.

"I know that Jesus Christ teaches us that love is the most important essence of life. So, I am thankful to know this and to love my birth family, my chosen spiritual family, as well as the human family, and to be kind and gracious to all."
Deborah Perdue

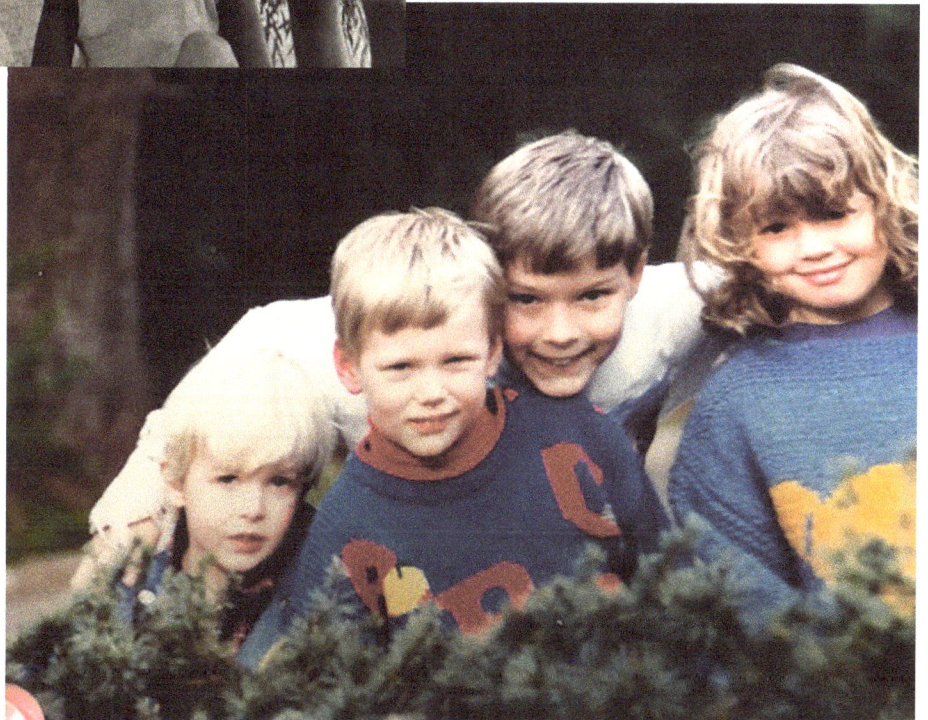

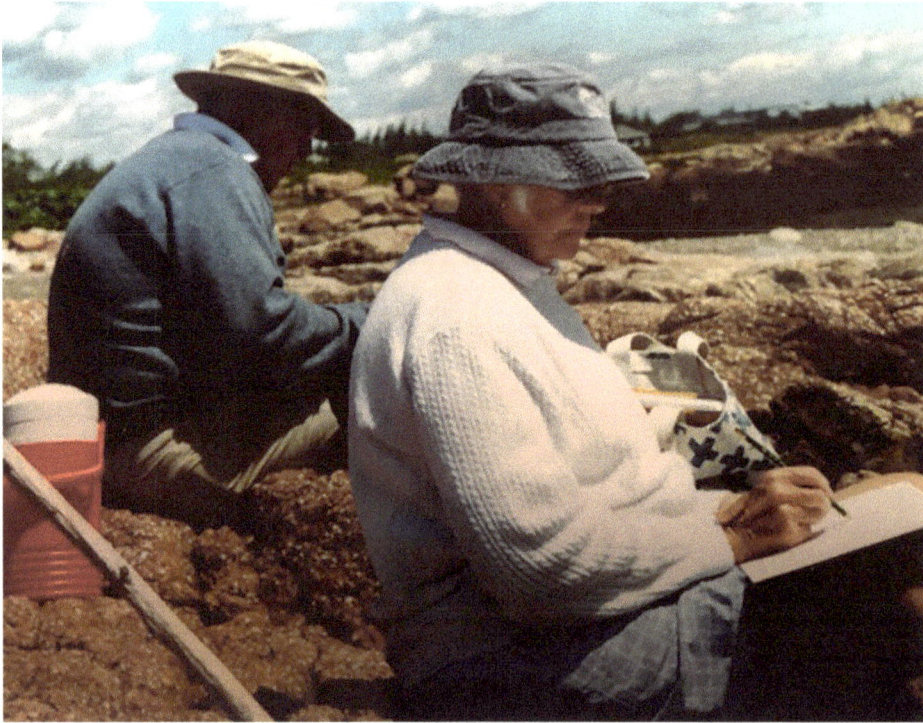

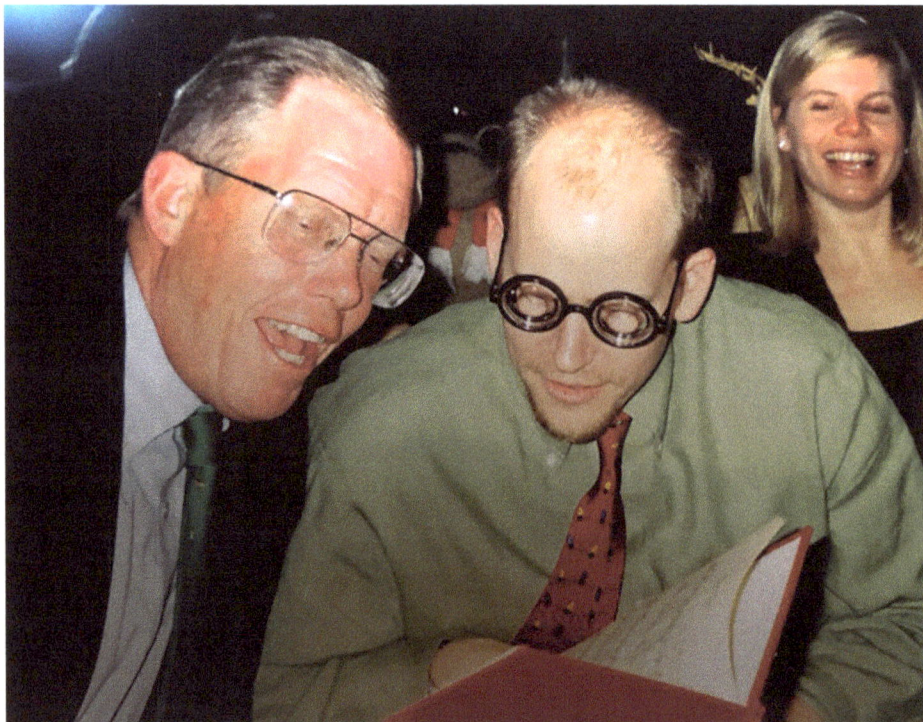

Been back from the normal world; lesson 5: when this dementia dude can't grasp a word or I forget where I am in the convo, folks, including me, think it's funny. But there is an unintended consequence. Normals are relieved. They see a symptom and can breathe easy. I am probably not faking dementia. Life is back in place and they don't have dementia. All is well in the world.

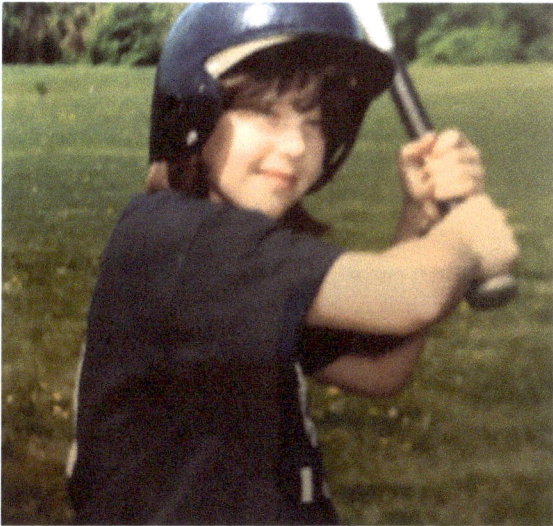

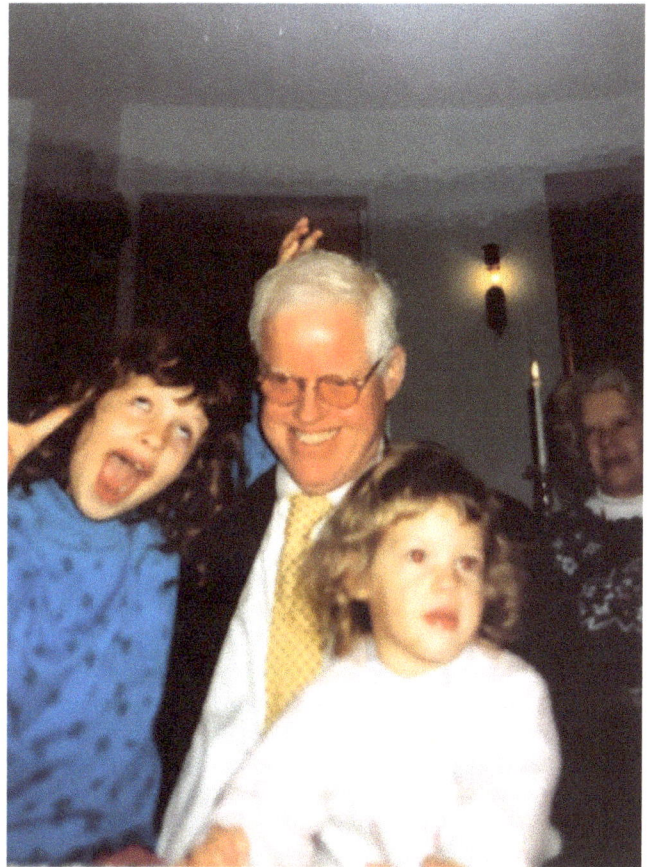

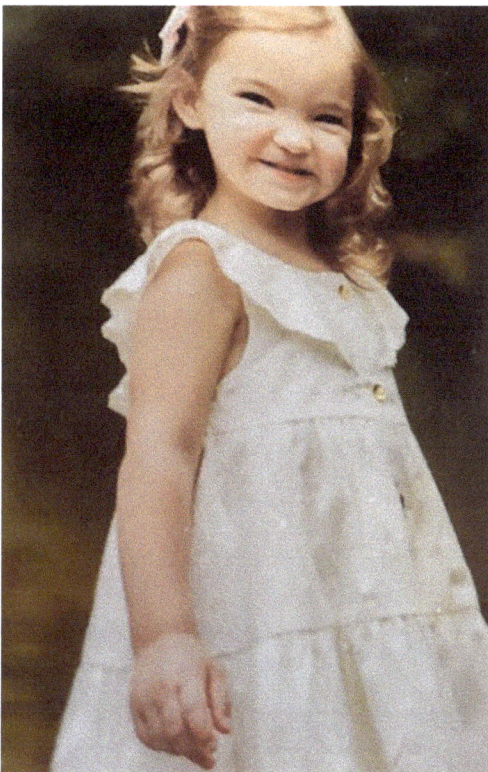

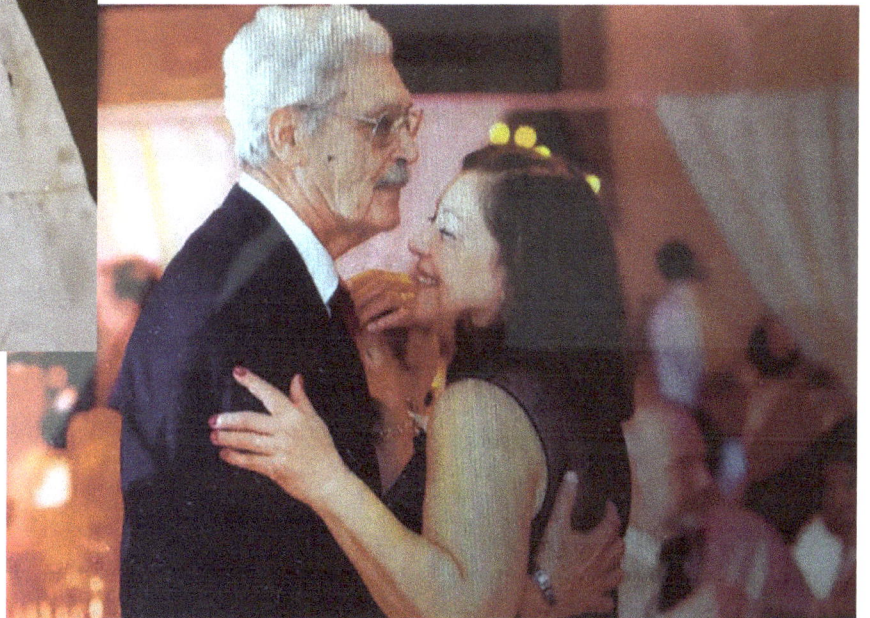

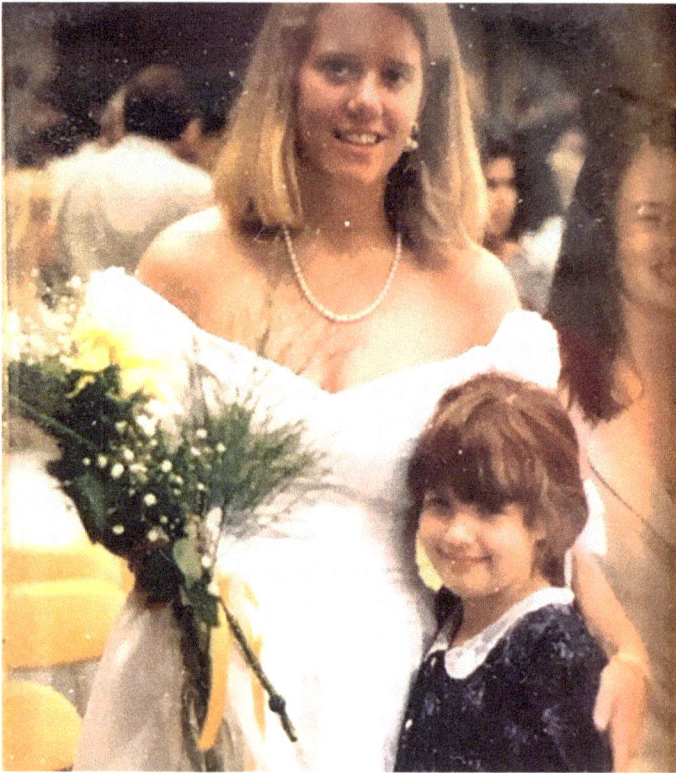
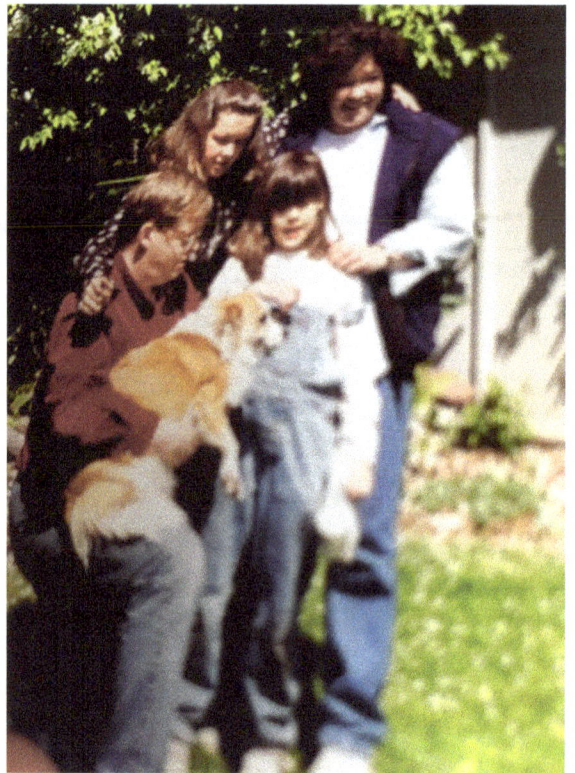
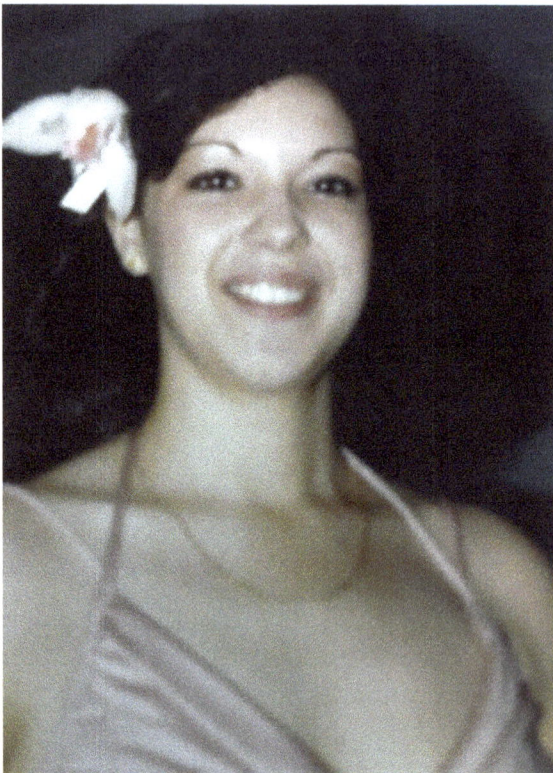
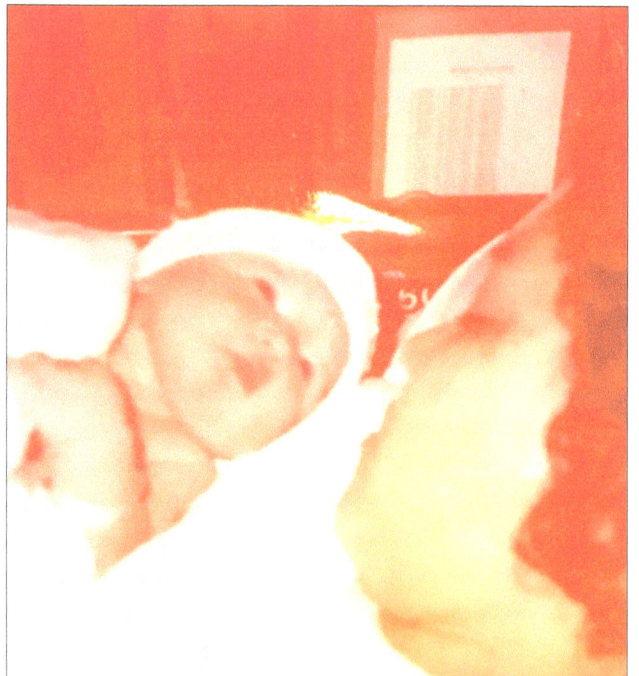

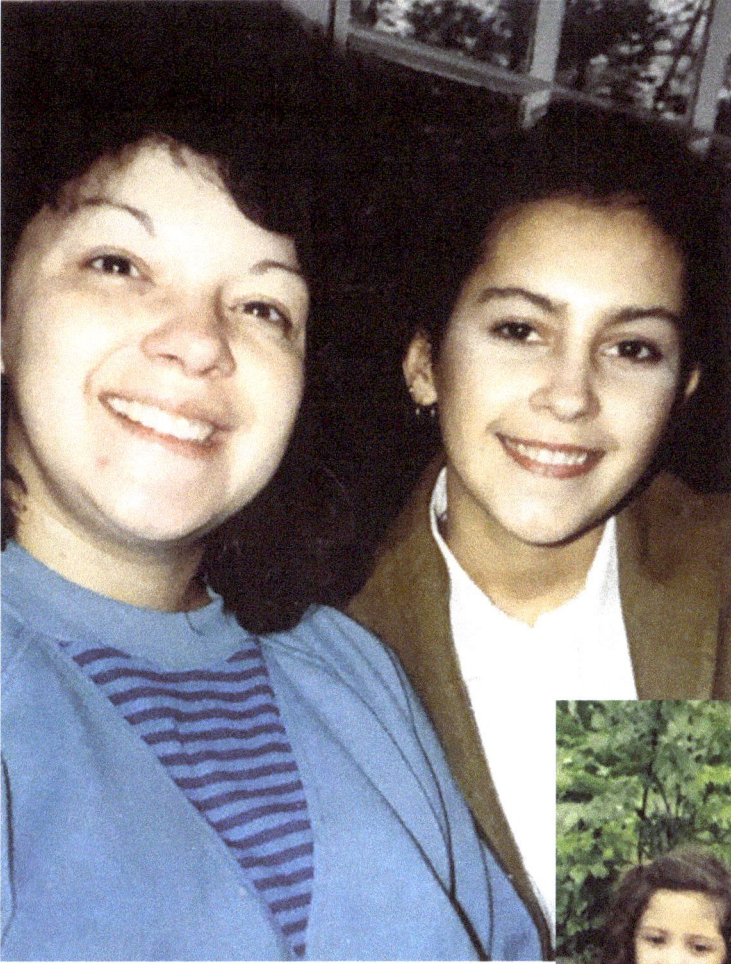

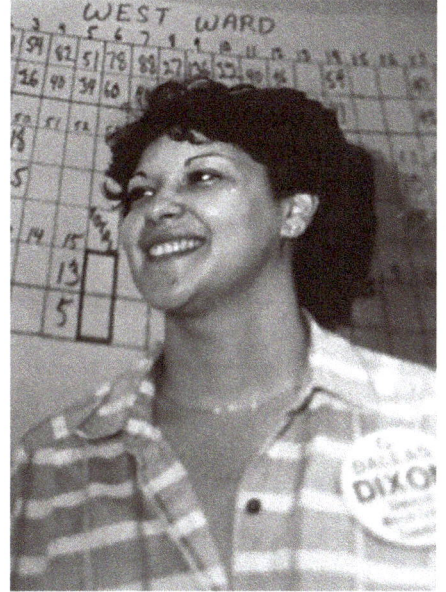

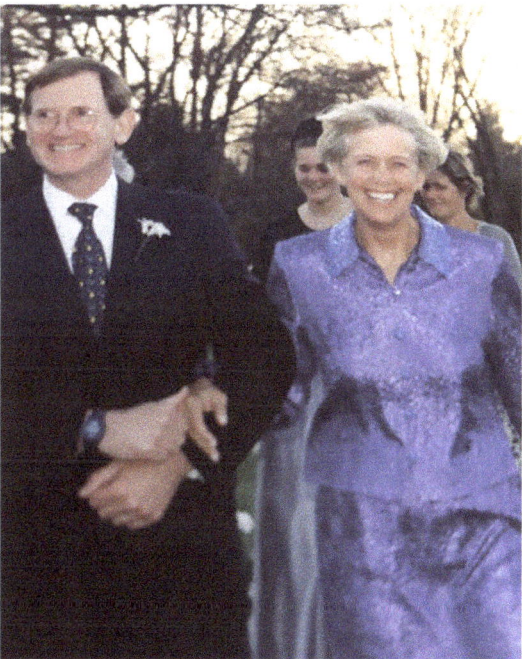

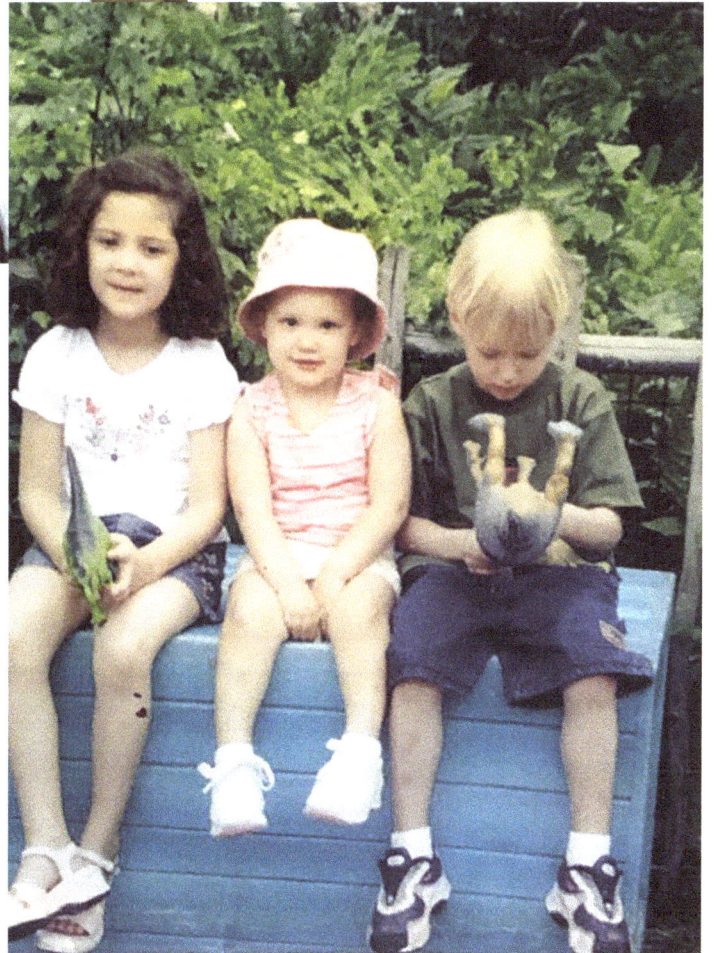

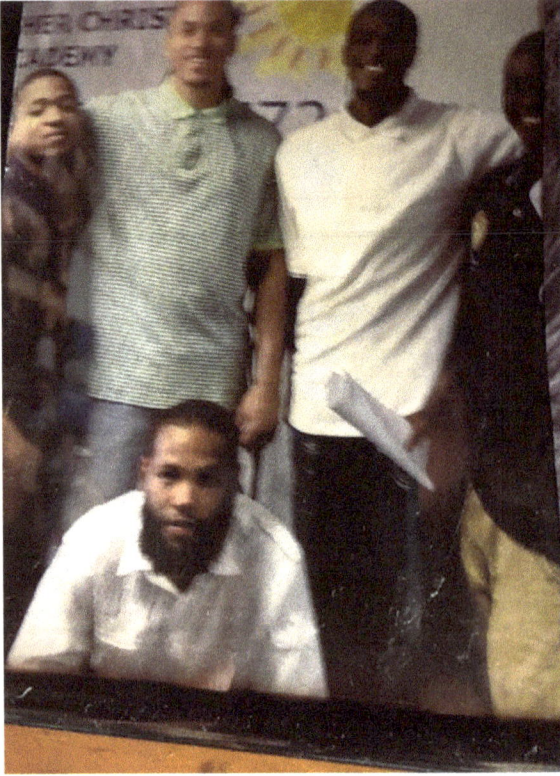

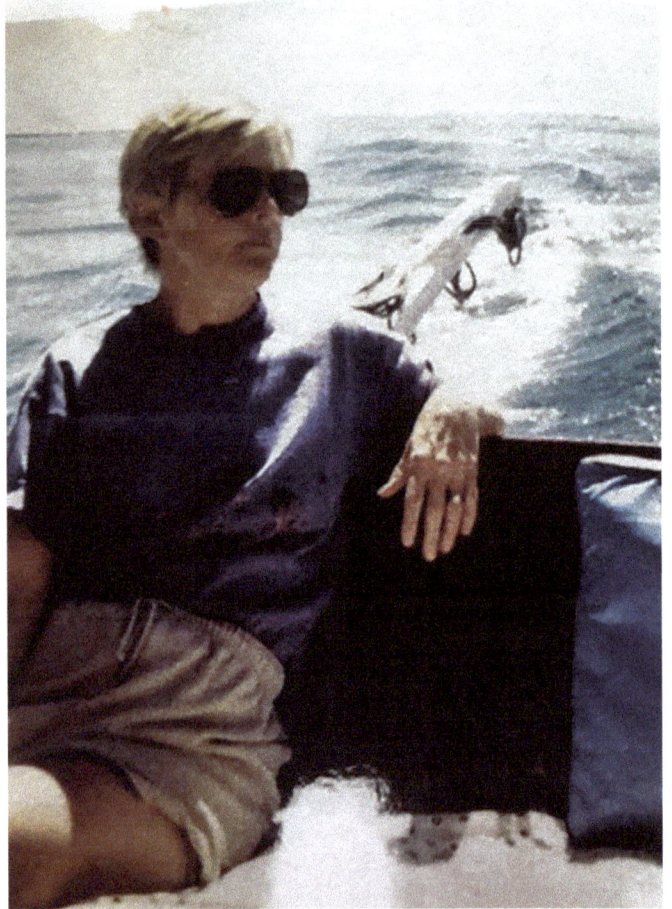

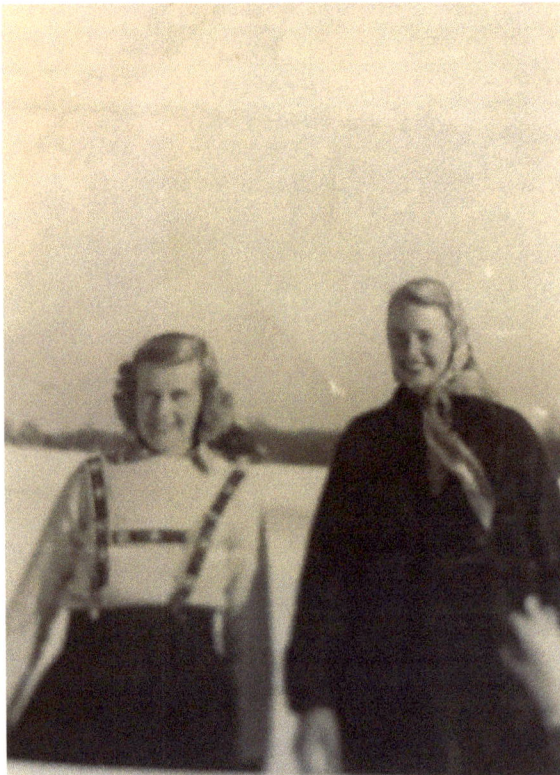

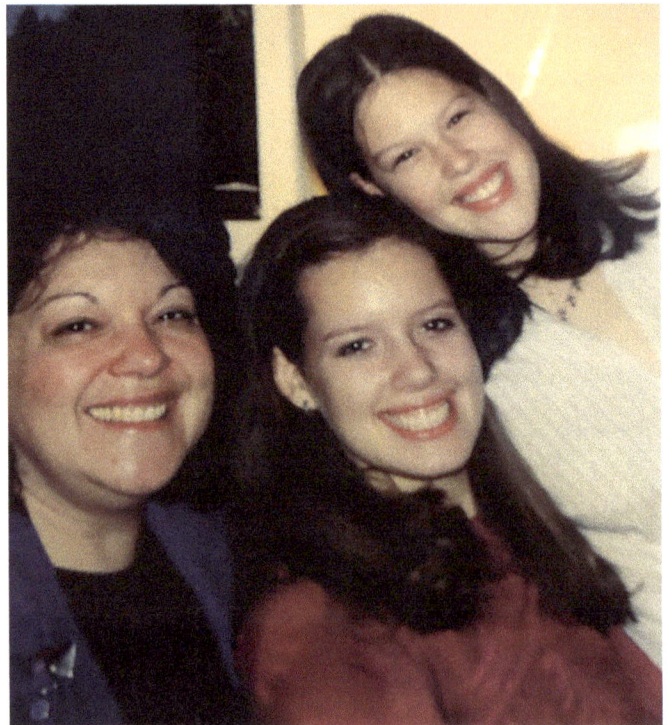

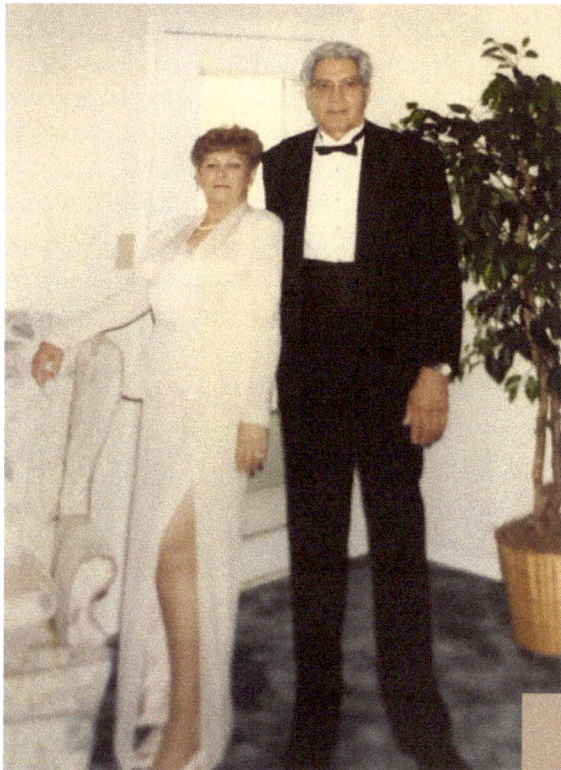

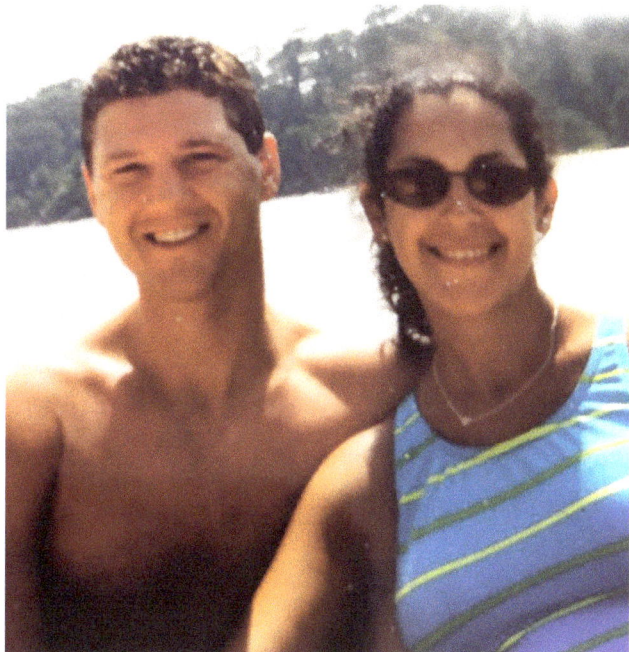

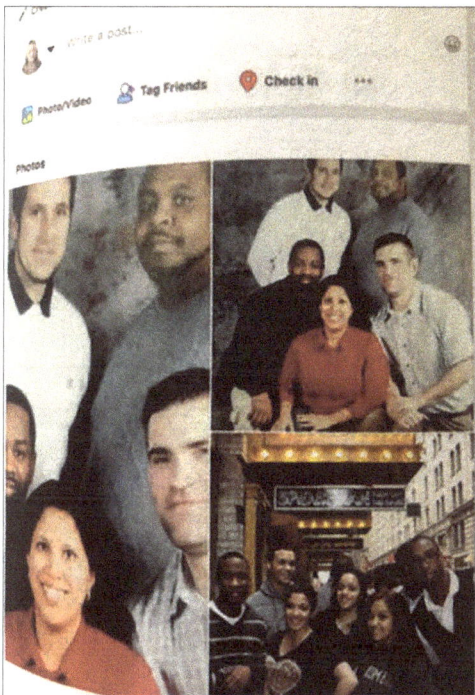

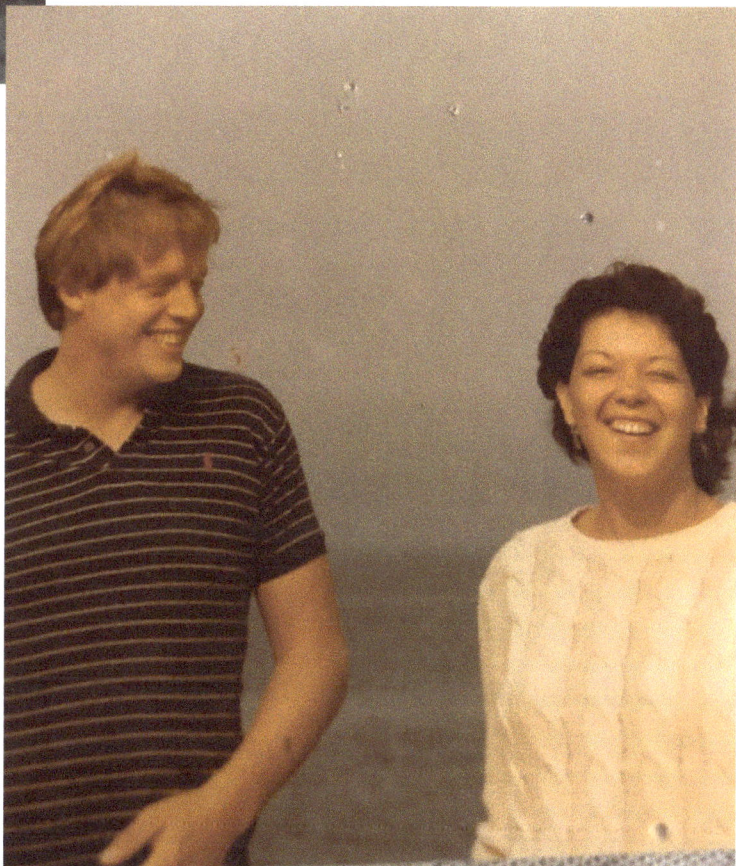

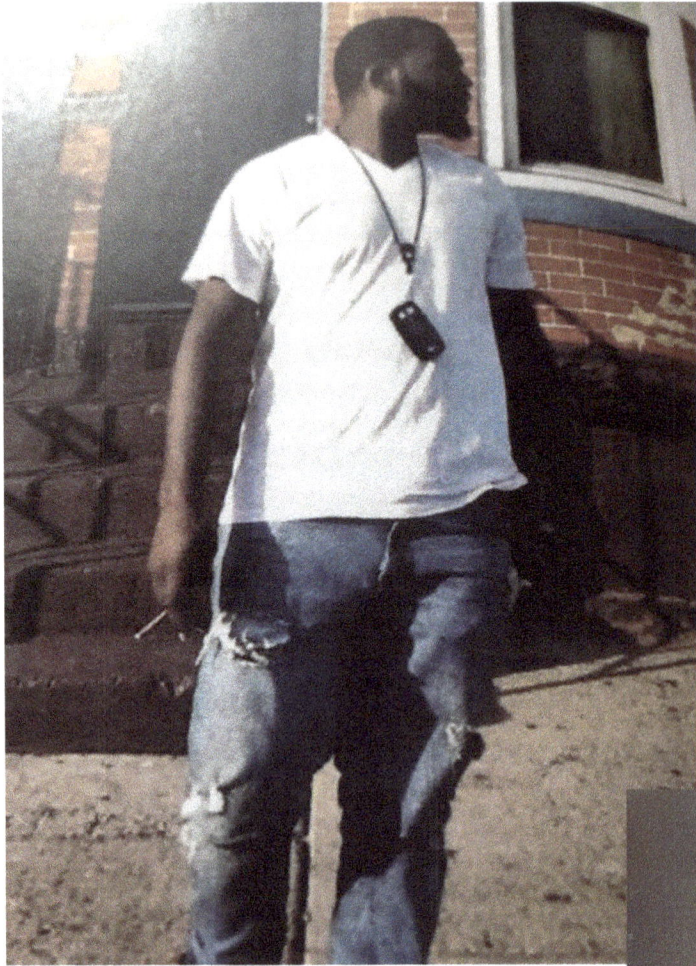
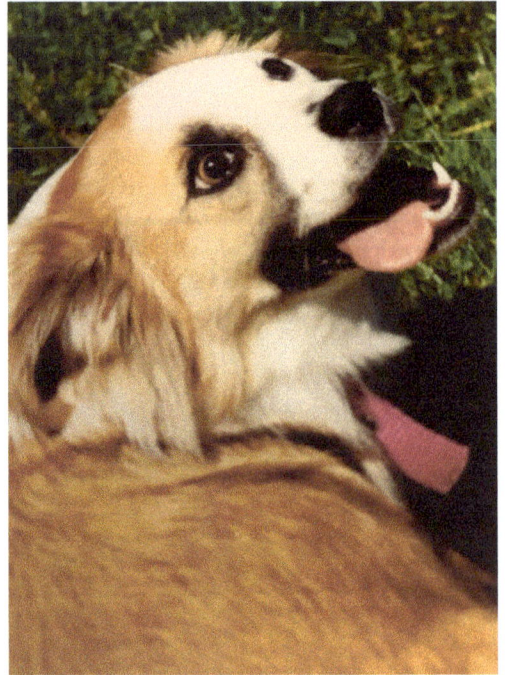
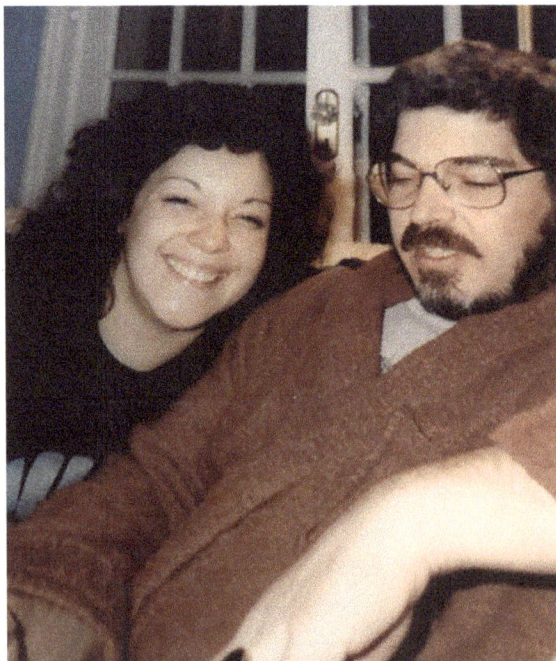
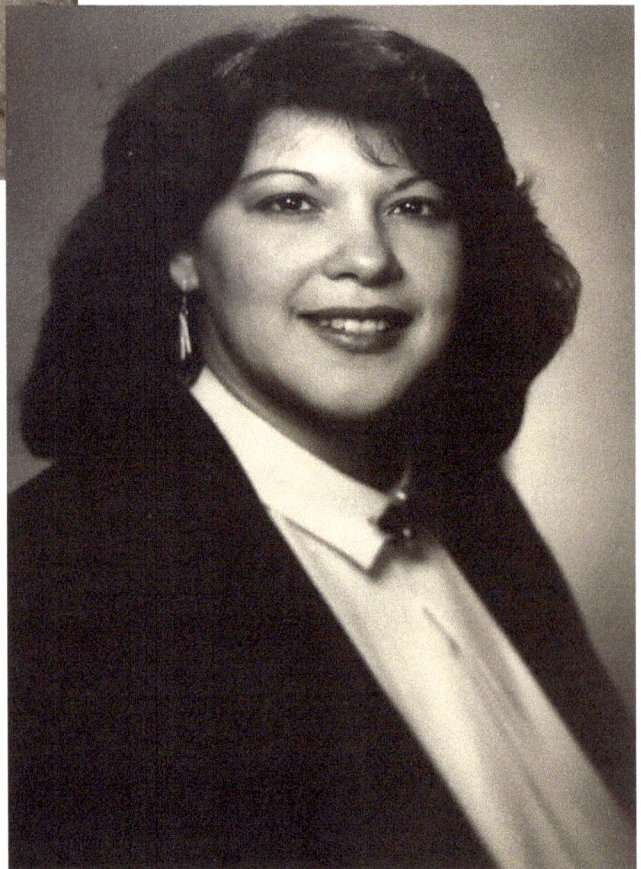

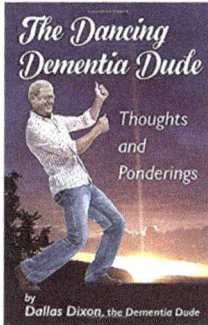

The Dancing Dementia Dude: Thoughts and Ponderings

by Dallas Dixon | Mar 30, 2020

Paperback

$6⁰⁰

FREE Delivery by **Fri, Sep 3** for Prime
members

More Buying Choices
$5.99 (2 used & new offers)

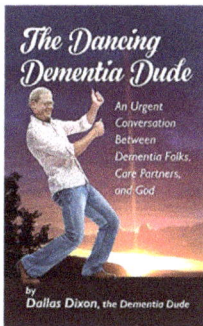

The Dancing Dementia Dude: An Urgent Conversation Between Dementia F

by Dallas Dixon | Mar 12, 2017

★★★★☆ ⌄ 4

Kindle

$5⁰⁰ ~~$20.00~~

Available instantly

Paperback

$20⁰⁰

✓prime FREE Delivery **Mon, Aug 30**

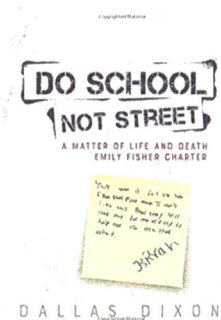

Do School Not Street

by Dallas Dixon | Oct 10, 2018

Paperback

$49⁵⁰

✓prime FREE Delivery **Mon, Aug 30**